# Neuropsychological Rehabilitation

T0383374

# Neuropsychological Rehabilitation
## Principles and Applications

*Edited by*

## Jamuna Rajeswaran

*Associate Professor and Consultant*
*Clinical Neuropsychology Unit*
*Department of Clinical Psychology*
*National Institute of Mental Health and Neurosciences*
*(NIMHANS)*
*Bangalore, Karnataka, India*

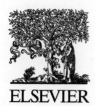

ELSEVIER    AMSTERDAM • BOSTON • HEIDELBERG • LONDON • NEW YORK • OXFORD
PARIS • SAN DIEGO • SAN FRANCISCO • SINGAPORE • SYDNEY • TOKYO

Elsevier
32 Jamestown Road, London NW1 7BY
225 Wyman Street, Waltham, MA 02451, USA

First edition 2013

**Notices**
Knowledge and best practice in this field are constantly changing. As new research and experience broaden our understanding, changes in research methods, professional practices, or medical treatment may become necessary.

Practitioners and researchers must always rely on their own experience and knowledge in evaluating and using any information, methods, compounds, or experiments described herein. In using such information or methods they should be mindful of their own safety and the safety of others, including parties for whom they have a professional responsibility.

To the fullest extent of the law, neither the Publisher nor the authors, contributors, or editors, assume any liability for any injury and/or damage to persons or property as a matter of products liability, negligence or otherwise, or from any use or operation of any methods, products, instructions, or ideas contained in the material herein.

**British Library Cataloguing-in-Publication Data**
A catalog record for this book is available from the British Library

**Library of Congress Cataloging-in-Publication Data**
A catalog record for this book is available from the Library of Congress

ISBN: 978-0-323-28248-2

For information on all Elsevier publications
visit our website at store.elsevier.com

This book has been manufactured using Print On Demand technology. Each copy is produced to order and is limited to black ink. The online version of this book will show color figures where appropriate.

Working together to grow
libraries in developing countries

www.elsevier.com | www.bookaid.org | www.sabre.org

ELSEVIER     BOOK AID International     Sabre Foundation

# Contents

# List of contributors

**C.N. Bennett**
Clinical Neuropsychology Unit, Department of Clinical Psychology, National Institute of Mental Health and Neurosciences (NIMHANS), Bangalore, Karnataka, India

**B.N. Gangadhar**
Department of Psychiatry, National Institute of Mental Health and Neurosciences (NIMHANS), Bangalore, Karnataka, India

**S. Hegde**
Cognitive Psychology Unit, Centre for Cognition and Human Excellence, National Institute of Mental Health and Neurosciences (NIMHANS), Bangalore, Karnataka, India

**H. Kashyap**
Clinical Neuropsychologist and researcher, Melbourne Neuropsychiatry Centre, National Neuroscience Facility, University of Melbourne, Australia.

**J. Keshav Kumar**
Neuropsychology Unit, Department of Clinical Psychology, National Institute of Mental Health and Neurosciences (NIMHANS), Bangalore, Karnataka, India

**C.R. Mukundan**
Scientific Adviser, Axxonet System Technologies, Research Institute of Gujarat Forensic Sciences University, Bangalore, Karnataka, India

**A. Nehra**
Department of Clinical Neuropsychology, Neurosciences Centre, All India Institute of Medical Sciences, New Delhi, India

**A. Raguram**
Department of Clinical Psychology, National Institute of Mental Health and Neurosciences (NIMHANS), Bangalore, Karnataka, India

**K. Rajakumari**
Clinical Neuropsychology Unit, Department of Clinical Psychology, National Institute of Mental Health and Neurosciences (NIMHANS), Bangalore, Karnataka, India

**J. Rajeswaran**
Clinical Neuropsychology Unit, Department of Clinical Psychology, National Institute of Mental Health and Neurosciences (NIMHANS), Bangalore, Karnataka, India

**S.L. Rao**
Cognitive Psychology Unit, Centre for Cognition and Human Excellence, National Institute of Mental Health and Neurosciences (NIMHANS), Bangalore, Karnataka, India

**D. Sadana**
Clinical Neuropsychology Unit, Department of Clinical Psychology, National Institute of Mental Health and Neurosciences (NIMHANS), Bangalore, Karnataka, India

**A. Sadasivan**
Samvidh Psychological Services, Bangalore, Karnataka, India

**E.A. Shereena**
Clinical Neuropsychology Unit, Department of Clinical Psychology, National Institute of Mental Health and Neuro Sciences (NIMHANS), Bangalore, Karnataka, India

**P.M. Sudhir**
Behavioral Medicine Unit, Department of Clinical Psychology, National Institute of Mental Health and Neurosciences (NIMHANS), Bangalore, Karnataka, India

**S. Thomas**
Clinical Neuropsychology Unit, Department of Clinical Psychology, National Institute of Mental Health and Neurosciences (NIMHANS), Bangalore, Karnataka, India

# 1 Neuropsychological Rehabilitation: Need and Scope

## J. Rajeswaran, C.N. Bennett, E.A. Shereena

Clinical Neuropsychology Unit, Department of Clinical Psychology,
National Institute of Mental Health and Neurosciences (NIMHANS),
Bangalore, Karnataka, India

*Last year I had a stroke. It left me in bad shape. I had to teach myself how to walk and talk all over again. It was a long hard fight. My speech is not perfect but I'm getting there.*

**Dick Clark, American businessman, stroke survivor**

## The Miracle of the Human Brain—The Basis for Neuropsychological Rehabilitation

We are all well familiar with the touching story of Paul Bach-y-Rita, one of the most influential theorists of neural plasticity. It is well known that Paul Bach-y-Rita was greatly influenced by his father Pedro's miraculous recovery following a severely debilitating stroke. Paul's brother George Bach-y-Rita employed some very unconventional methods to rehabilitate his father and succeeded well beyond anybody's imagination. Pedro Bach-y-Rita recovered enough to take on full-time teaching and died 7 years after a heart attack in a mountain-climbing expedition. The story was far from over with Pedro's death. Postautopsy reports indicate that approximately 97% of the cerebrospinal nerves were destroyed. Needless to say, this was a huge blow to the localization theory, which states that brain structures are hardwired to perform a limited set of functions.

The enchantment of neuropsychological rehabilitation (NR), therefore, rightfully lies in the marvel of the brain itself. The brain is an organ that continues to remain an enigma. While the mysteries of the brain are slowly but surely being unravelled by advances in cognitive neurosciences, one can argue that we are no closer to the absolute truth.

Neuropsychological Rehabilitation-Principles and Applications.
DOI: http://dx.doi.org/10.1016/B978-0-12-416046-0.00001-8

## Definition and Introduction

NR is concerned with the amelioration of cognitive, emotional, psychosocial, and behavioral deficits caused by an insult to the brain [1]. NR, needless to say, has made its mark as a vital aspect of intervention for brain-related dysfunction. At the outset, it must be stated that the authors do not believe in the existence of a standard NR procedure. While this particular statement made may seem debatable, maybe even controversial, the need for it to be stated is that the authors take on a purely phenomenological approach to rehabilitation. While it is generally agreed that there are certain basic principles of rehabilitation, the manner of rehabilitation depends on several factors. The course of intervention is decided based not only on the diagnosis of the patient but also on the individual patient's age, premorbid functioning, education, background, etc., and the therapist's innovative skill in developing tasks to address these functions. Also to be kept in mind are the behavioral, social, and emotional ramifications of the dysfunction in the patient's life as well as in the lives of those interacting with the patient.

NR has application in several brain-related conditions such as traumatic brain injuries (TBIs), tumors, cerebrovascular accidents, anoxia, brain-related infectious conditions, neurodegenerative conditions, and psychiatric disorders. The nature of brain-related pathophysiology is different in these various conditions, and the thrust of the rehabilitation procedures needs to be modified accordingly. Although the basic outlook of rehabilitation in these conditions tends to be varied, the basic principles of NR remain constant. However, it must be stated that among all these conditions, it is the area of TBI rehabilitation that appears to be most well researched. The reasons for this are yet unclear. Possible explanations may include the extreme burden of health care, loss of productive years of the individual, and loss of manpower resources that such injuries entail. It may also be due to the increasing incidence of such injuries in adolescents and young adults. In India alone, TBI has an incidence of 150/100,000 and a mortality rate of 20/100,000 [2].

While cognitive dysfunction forms the core aspect of intervention, a neuropsychologist's role is not simply limited to the remediation of cognitive deficits. NR is also interested in addressing the emotional disturbances associated with the disorder, behavioral dysfunctions, and the lacuna in social functioning subsequent to brain dysfunction.

## Neuropsychological Assessment—A Precursor to the Development of a Sound Neuropsychological Rehabilitation Program

The importance of neuropsychological assessment in planning intervention modules can never be overemphasized. Neuropsychological assessment is an interface between neurology, psychiatry, and psychology, and it represents various convergent disciplines, including neuroanatomy, neurochemistry, neurophysiology, cognitive neuroscience, and neuropharmachology. Neuropsychological assessment measures encompass a wide range of tests, beginning with 10-minute screening tools and extending to exhaustive batteries that last for a few hours. Both qualitative and quantitative measures form an important part of neuropsychological assessment. Significant aspects of neuropsychological testing include assessing the mental state of the individual and testing the functions of the brain based on its known physiology. Neuropsychological tests are scientific, standardized on normal individuals. Tests have been designed to assess sensory input, attention and concentration, learning and memory, language functions, spatial and manipulatory ability, executive functions, and motor output [3].

The neuropsychological assessment provides diagnostic information about the nature and extent of cognitive dysfunction following various neurological, neurosurgical, and psychiatric conditions. In addition to its utility as a diagnostic tool, assessment findings play a vital role in planning NR. Hence, the aim of cognitive rehabilitation is to address cognitive dysfunction. Apart from this, neuropsychological intervention also attempts to address the emotional, social, and psychological implications of brain pathology.

Several cognitive deficits have been associated with TBI. Cicerone [4] reports deficits in attention and difficulty in dual task demands even with patients with mild TBI. McDowell et al. [5] confirm working memory deficits in individuals with TBI using other dual task paradigms. Brooks et al. [6] report significant differences in frontal lobe executive functions in individuals with TBI in comparison with control subjects. Difficulties in memory have also been reported. In a study by Hamm et al. [7], deficits in performance on the Morris water maze was found to be diminished in rats that had sustained brain injury.

Other aspects of neuropsychological functioning include assessment of stress, depression, anxiety, behavior analyses, social functioning, and quality of life. Addressing these factors helps in assessing outcome and enables better prognostication. A well-administered neuropsychological assessment not only prognosticates but also helps in the development of specific goals for rehabilitation.

# Theories of Neuropsychological Intervention

A good NR program requires a foundation of strong theoretical frameworks.

## The Role of Neuronal Plasticity

The environment can alter the organization of the normal and injured brain through the mechanism of brain plasticity [8]. Neuronal plasticity refers to the adaptation of the brain as a result of several factors that may independently or through interaction produce changes in the brain. Neural plasticity may occur as a part of normal developmental function, or it may be the result of a response to destroyed brain function due to brain injury. The environment plays an important role in brain plasticity. Enriched environments have been demonstrated to be associated with greater levels of dendritic growth, particularly in the hippocampus. This ability of the human brain to adapt itself, is what makes neurorehabilitation possible.

### The Role of Restitution, Substitution, and Compensation

In 1947, Zangwill (as cited in Wilson and Glisky [9]) described three processes of rehabilitation. The first, "restitution," describes a process of restoration of the lost or impaired function. The second, referred to as "substitution training," involves the replacement of impaired functions by alternate strategies that prove to be functional. This may also involve the reorganization of cortical networks associated with the task. The third, which is described as "compensation," requires an artificial source that typically requires more effort and time .

### The Role of Diaschisis and the Unmasking of Latent Neural Pathways

Diaschisis refers to the excitatory and inhibitory effects following brain injury that affect areas remote to the site of injury. These effects were used to explain the sequelae following the injury. Although diaschisis was originally used to explain the deficits following head injury, it may indeed work as a blessing in disguise. In a normal uninjured brain, there exist certain pathways that are ineffective and inactive. Diaschisis may indeed inhibit this original suppression thereby rendering these alternate pathways functional [10].

## Major Influences and Recent Advances in the Development of Rehabilitative Neuropsychology

To begin our understanding of the present need and scope of NR, it is necessary to frame the current trends in the perspective of the past of NR and where its current practices stem from.

The earliest recorded information we possess on localization of function in the brain is contained in the Edwin Smith Surgical Papyrus. The copy acquired by Smith in Luxor in 1862 is thought to date from the seventeenth century BC, while orthographic and other evidence would place its origin some thousand years earlier, somewhere between 2500 and 3000 BC. It contains the earliest known anatomical, physiological, and pathological descriptions and has been described as the earliest known scientific document. The papyrus contains reports of some 48 cases of observation and description of treatment of actual cases, many of them suffering from traumatic lesions of various parts of the body, including the head and the neck. Of the 48 cases, the first 8 deals directly with injuries to the head and the brain [11].

Other important influences include the proposition of the Hebbian law that succinctly states that "what fires together wires together." The original theory reads as follows: "When an axon of cell A is near enough to excite cell B or repeatedly or persistently takes part in firing it, some growth process or metabolic change takes place in one or both cells such that A's efficiency, as one of the cells firing B, is increased." The activity of one neuron that influences another neuron thereby forms the basis of neuronal plasticity through long-term potentiation and long-term depression.

Attempts at rehabilitation can be traced back to Paul Broca's attempt to enable a patient who had reading difficulty [12]. Efforts at rehabilitation can also be attributed to Shepherd Franz, who was known for his work on motor learning in patients with hemiparesis and therapeutic approach with aphasic patients. The centers for rehabilitation set up in Europe during the world wars also played a vital role in unfolding of the rehabilitation as we understand it now. Goldstein's documentation of treatment of disorders of speech, reading, and writing, the effects of fatigue on performance, and the unique manner in which each patient is to be treated also deserve a special mention [12]. The methods of assessment during the time of World War II resulting in a formal detailed neuropsychological profile can be credited to Russian psychologist Luria. The work of Ben-Yishay in the late 1970s and the 1980s also highlighted the importance of considering the interpersonal and social aspects of the patient in fostering reintegration into the social world [13].

Of course, we have progressed much since the Edwin Papyrus. Lesion and radiological studies have of course ascribed specific functions to specific locations. However, as mentioned earlier, the work by Bach-y-Rita and several others indicate that this is not so simple.

## Methods of Neuropsychological Rehabilitation

There has been a change in the perspective of intervention in the care of brain-related injuries. While initial perspectives focused on acute management and intensive medical care targeting basic survival, later approaches appear to address the outcomes of the injury in terms of basic functioning and quality of life.

It has been found that attention remediation is effective in improving deficits of focused, sustained, and divided attention [14]. The use of hospital-based cognitive retraining in individuals with impairments in ideational fluency, abstraction, working memory, verbal and visual memory, and information processing has been well demonstrated. The findings showed reduction in symptoms and enhancement of cognitive functions and well-being in patients with TBI when compared with a control group [15]. Computer-based retraining programs are used apart from the traditional methods of retraining, and current advances include use of computer-based retraining techniques and the use of pagers and other memory aids [9]. Also taking its place among the recent developments is EEG neurofeedback training. EEG neurofeedback, also popularly known as biofeedback, is used to modify amplitude, frequency, and even coherency of one's own brain waves using operation conditioning methods [16].

The efficacy of neurofeedback intervention in TBI is fairly well established. Improvement has been reported in mild TBI after 20 treatment sessions of neurofeedback intervention and cognitive retraining [17]. Neurofeedback therapy used to enhance sensorimotor rhythm and train for beta while suppressing theta is a promising intervention technique in mild head injury [18]. The use of neurofeedback in the early stages of brain injury, reporting the remediation of attention difficulties in closed head injury patients, has also been discussed in the context of spontaneous recovery [19]. Neurofeedback has been used to improve physical balance, incontinence, and swallowing in four cases, suggesting that the intervention technique holds much promise in conditions of the elderly, stroke, brain injury, primary nocturnal enuresis, and peak performance training, where balance is imperative [20]. Memory and learning improvement have also been found after the use of neurofeedback intervention [21,22].

# Need for Intervention

By 2020, the incidence of TBI is projected to increase worldwide. The death rate is estimated to rise from 5.1 to 8.4 million. The most important cause of death up to 45 years of age will be TBI [23]. These projected figures have serious implications. Every year approximately 1.7 million people sustain a TBI. Among them, 52,000 die, 275,000 are hospitalized, and 1.365 million are treated and discharged from emergency services [24]. Stroke is the third most common cause of death and the leading cause of serious, long-term disability in the United States [25]. Stroke can occur at any age; nearly one-fourth of strokes occur in people under the age of 65 [26]. Needless to say, the cost of health-care places a major strain on any economy. Also, with the advancement of medical science, mortality rates are on the decline, thereby increasing the need of rehabilitating the survivors. It poses a great challenge and burden for health-care professionals. Therefore, it becomes vital for medical and allied science professionals to develop efficacious preventive and intervention programs to deal with this seemingly intractable predicament.

# Vital Issues and Current Trends

NR has seen several changes during its course. Some important aspects of rehabilitation that are currently being addressed are discussed below.

## Caregiver Burden: Giving Till It Hurts

*Take a deep breath and really acknowledge all that you have been doing.*
*You are an unsung hero and it is important*
*that you accept the beauty of who you are in this moment.*
*… look into the mirror into your eyes*
*and honor "yourself" for all you have been doing and will continue to do.*
*National Organization for Empowering Caregivers*

Caregivers and the families of the patient play an important role in the rehabilitation of individuals with neuropsychological dysfunction. Illness can be extremely debilitating, threatening the structure of the entire family system, and creating severe distress. Cognitive, emotional, and behavioral difficulties and personality changes such as anger, irritability, poor frustration tolerance, and dependency cause the greatest distress among family members and caregivers. The role of the caregiver and patient may be reversed; for instance, the caregiver may need to take on financial responsibilities, which further burdens this fragile system. In 1998, Marsh et al. [27] reported that among individuals with TBI, physical impairment, the number of behavioral problems, and social isolation were the strongest predictors of caregiver burden. An effective NR program addresses the needs not only of the patient but also of those who are closely allied with the patient.

The role of the caregiver also becomes important in the rehabilitation process as the caregiver begins to act as a co-therapist. A successful NR program empowers caregivers to meet desired goals. Like a ripple created by a pebble thrown into a still lake, the rehabilitation specialist's influence must extend beyond the immediate target. However, in practice, it may not be as easy to foster the active participation of caregivers. Strained relationships resulting from the trauma, aggravation of existing stressors, disruption of family roles, and ineffective communication patterns all contribute to hindering treatment. Addressing caregiver burden therefore becomes an important aspect of a successful neuropsychological program.

## Rehabilitation of Pediatric Populations

*It is never too late to have a happy childhood.*

*Tom Robbins*

Childhood is a crucial period in the development of the human brain. Although the brain is believed to be plastic throughout its lifetime, it is during childhood through adolescence that the brain is known to mature the most. Acquired brain injuries such as TBI, Central Nervous System (CNS) infections, meningitis, encephalitis, stroke, and hypoxia/anoxia can lead to significant cognitive and behavioral disabilities. Although children with focal brain injuries acquire many age-related skills, evidence suggests that "crowding effects" in children, wherein one area of the brain takes over the functions of the affected area, leads to a general decrease in neurobehavioral function. Age at the time of injury is very crucial. The earlier the injury, the smaller the store of learned knowledge and skills and the greater the likelihood of global impairment [28,29].

The concept of plasticity differs in the child population, as brain regions do not have clearly defined functions. Early injury disrupts the acquisition of basic skills required for later healthy development. Involving parents in the rehabilitation process and providing psychoeducation is essential. Contact with school authorities and providing them with inputs on teaching methods suited for the child with specific deficits is also an integral part of the rehabilitation process.

NR involves the recovery of lost functions; in pediatric care, it may also include the acquisition of functions not previously acquired. Research studies on rehabilitation of children are few and lack rigorous control conditions. Cognitive retraining, EEG neurofeedback training, and other computerized training techniques are widely used and have been found to be effective. Despite the high vulnerability of the immature brain, the joy of working with a pediatric population lies in the advantage of neural plasticity being at its greatest during this period.

## Static Versus Progressive Conditions

There is evidence to suggest that cognitive retraining can be beneficial even in neurodegenerative conditions. There is also some indication that these gains can be maintained beyond the final session [30]. There has been, however, some controversy regarding the use of cognitive retraining techniques in progressive conditions. While there has been some indication that it may hasten progressive decline, this view remains largely unsupported.

## Medico-Legal Cases

Identifying malingering and quantifying the extent of disability has become an important source of concern in neurorehabilitation. Health-care expenses pose a constraint on the economy of any nation. Compensation and monetary benefits are one reason for malingering. Other reasons may include avoidance of penalties. Malingering, of course, should be distinguished from dissociation experiences, which require to be treated from a psychological perspective.

## Setting Up a Rehabilitation Center

*The only thing worse than being blind is having sight but no vision.*

*Helen Keller*

Setting up a rehabilitation institute for remediation of brain-related dysfunction is no simple feat. Needless to say, rehabilitation requires a committed group of multidisciplinary specialists from medicine, surgery, physiotherapy, occupational therapy, speech therapy, social work, neuropsychology, and other allied services. Creating a rehabilitation facility cannot simply be a conglomeration of various specialities; it requires vision. It is that sense of purpose in enhancing the patient's ultimate well-being that sows the seeds for the establishment of a well-endowed rehabilitation program. Apart from this, the visionary must also have strong administrative skills to bring to fruition the plan envisioned in his/her mind. (S)he must be able to envision both immediate and long-term goals of the program while establishing a system that is both efficient and self-sustaining.

# Conclusion

*It seems to me that unless you or someone very close to you has had a bad head injury, you really can't fathom it. You have no concept of what it is all about. It was so difficult for my whole family, not just me.*

*American country music singer and brain injury survivor*

The truth of the matter is that rehabilitation is a very difficult business. It can be challenging for the therapist and at times can be a draining experience. It becomes important at such times to take a step back and reconsider one's goals. However, while it may be challenging it also presents itself as a rewarding experience. The therapist is not simply a giver but learns and changes through the process. The need of rehabilitation having been firmly established gives this discipline scope for unimaginable growth. While it is hard to determine where the wind blows for NR, given its growth in leaps and bounds, it can be safely stated that the wind blows strongly and surely.

# References

[1] Wilson, B. A. (2008). Neuropsychological rehabilitation. *Annual Review of Clinical Psychology, 4*, 141–162.

[2] Gururaj, G., Kolluri., S. V. R., Chandramouli, B. A, Subbakrishna, D. K., & Kraus, J. F. (2005). *Traumatic brain injury* (Vol. 61). Bangalore: National Institute of Mental Health & Neuro Sciences.

[3] Gregory, R. J. (2000). *Psychological testing: History, principles, and applications.* Boston: Allyn and Bacon.

[4] Cicerone, K. D. (1996). Attention deficits and dual task demands after mild traumatic brain injury. *Brain Injury, 10*(2), 79–90.

[5] McDowell, S., Whyte, J., & D'Esposito, M. (1997). Working memory impairments in traumatic brain injury: Evidence from a dual-task paradigm. *Neuropsychologia, 35*(10), 1341–1353.

[6] Brooks, J., Fos, L. A., Greve, K. W., & Hammond, J. S. (1999). Assessment of executive function in patients with mild traumatic brain injury. *Journal of Trauma, 46*(1), 159–163.

[7] Hamm, R. J., Dixon, C. E., Gbadebo, D. M., Singha, A. K., Jenkins, L. W., Lyeth, B. G., et al. (1992). Cognitive deficits following traumatic brain injury produced by controlled cortical impact. *Journal of Neurotrauma, 9*(1), 11–20.

[8] Kolb, B., & Whishaw, I. Q. (2003). *Fundamentals of human neuropsychology.* New York: Worth Publishers.

[9] Wilson, B. A., & Glisky, E. L. (2009). *Memory rehabilitation: Integrating theory and practice.* New York: Guilford Press.

[10] Christensen, A. L., & Uzzell, B. P. (2000). *International handbook of neuropsychological rehabilitation.* New York: Kluwer Academic/Plenum Publishers.

[11] Darby, D., & Walsh, K. W. (2005). *Walsh's neuropsychology: A clinical approach.* Edinburgh: Elsevier Churchill Livingstone.

[12] Wilson, B. A., & Zangwill, O. L. (2003). *Neuropsychological rehabilitation: Theory and practice.* Exton, Pennsylvania: Swets & Zeitlinger Publishers.

[13] D'Amato, R. C., & Hartlage, L. C. (2008). *Essentials of neuropsychological assessment: Treatment planning for rehabilitation.* New York: Springer Publishing Company.

[14] Nag, S., & Rao, S. L. (1999). Remediation of attention deficits in head injury. *Neurology India, 47*(1), 32–39.

[15] Kumar, K., & Rao, S. L. (1999). *Cognitive retraining in traumatic brain injury.* Unpublished Thesis. Bangalore: NIMHANS.

[16] Thatcher, R. W., Moore, N., John, E. R., Duffy, F., Hughes, J. R., & Krieger, M. (1999). QEEG and traumatic brain injury: Rebuttal of the American Academy of

Neurology 1997 report by the EEG and Clinical Neuroscience Society. *Clinical Electroencephalography*, *30*(3), 94–98.

[17] Tinius, T. P., & Tinius, K. A. (2000). Changes after EEG biofeedback and cognitive retraining in adults with mild traumatic brain injury and attention deficit hyperactivity disorder. *Journal of Neurotherapy*, *4*(2), 27–43.

[18] Byers, A. P. J. (1995). Neurofeedback therapy for a mild head injury. *Journal of Neurotherapy*, *1*(1), 22–37.

[19] Keller, I. (2001). Neurofeedback therapy of attention deficits in patients with traumatic brain injury. *Journal of Neurotherapy*, *5*(1), 9–32.

[20] Hammond, D. C. (2006). Neurofeedback to improve physical balance, incontinence, and swallowing. *Journal of Neurotherapy*, *9*(1), 27–48.

[21] Thornton, K. E. (2000). Rehabilitation of memory functioning in brain injured subjects with EEG biofeedback. *Journal of Head Trauma Rehabilitation*, *15*(6), 1285–1296.

[22] Reddy, R. P., Jamuna, R., Bagavathula, I., & Kandavel, T. (2009). Neurofeedback training to enhance learning and memory in patient with traumatic brain injury: A single case study. *International Journal of Psychosocial Rehabilitation*, *14*(1), 21–22.

[23] Kiening, K., & Unterberg, A. (2007). Trauma care in Germany: A European perspective. *Clinical Neurosurgury*, *54*, 206–208.

[24] Faul, M. X. L., Wald, M. M., & Coronado, V. G. (2010). *Traumatic brain injury in the United States: Emergency department visits, hospitalizations, and deaths*. Atlanta, GA: Centers for Disease Control and Prevention NCfIPaC.

[25] Jack, V. T., Nardi, L., Fang, J., Liu, J., Khalid, L., & Johansen, H. (2009). National trends in rates of death and hospital admissions related to acute myocardial infarction, heart failure and stroke, 1994–2004. *Canadian Medical Association Journal*, June 23, 180.

[26] Tong, X., Kuklina, E. V., Gillespie, C., & George, M. G. (2011). Trends of acute ischemic stroke hospitalizations by age and gender in the United States, 1994–2007. *Paper presented on international stroke conference 2011*. Available from <http://www.abstractsonline.com>.

[27] Marsh, N. V., Kersel, D. A., Havill, J. H., & Sleigh, J. W. (1998). Caregiver burden at 1 year following severe traumatic brain injury. *Brain Injury*, *12*(12), 1045–1059.

[28] Dennis, M. (1999). *Childhood medical disorders and cognitive impairment: Biological risk, time*, development and reserve. In K. Yeates, & H. Taylor (Eds.), *Pediatric neuropsychology: Research, theory and practice* (pp. 3–22). New York: Guilford Press.

[29] Temple, C. (1997). *Developmental cognitive neuropsychology*. Hove, UK: Psychology Press.

[30] Clare, B. W., Carter, G., Hodges, J. R., & Adams, M. (2001). Long-term maintenance of treatment gains following a cognitive rehabilitation intervention in early dementia of Alzheimer type: A single case study. *Neuropsychological Rehabilitation*, *11*, 477–494.

# 2 Computerized Cognitive Retraining Programs for Patients Afflicted with Traumatic Brain Injury and Other Brain Disorders

C.R. Mukundan

Department of Clinical Psychology, National Institute of Mental Health and Neurosciences (NIMHANS), Bangalore, India

## Introduction

Neuropsychological rehabilitation is an important therapeutic program for the social and vocational remediation of patients who have suffered brain damage and consequent impairment in cognitive, emotional, and behavioral domains. Cognition refers to the mental processes of attending; selecting stimuli; their recognition, encoding, and transcoding; and storing and remembering information. Mentally holding onto such information and action plans for further processing may lead to problem solving and decision making based on which actions may be initiated and executed. Cognitive retraining is the method used for full or partial restoration of lost cognitive processing abilities, facilitating the patient's return to premorbid levels of cognitive functioning or helping them adapt to new social and occupational opportunities. Retraining and restoration of cognitive functions require an understanding of normal processing faculties in the brain, as established by scientific studies of these functions and their developmental patterns. Cognitive functions constitute interpretation of neural signals to information and using other capabilities for learning, storage, and retrieval of information. Billions of interconnected neurons and other cells in the brain support these functions. The neurons conduct and process neural signals, and groups of them in the neocortex are endowed with specific functional properties for carrying out processes that contribute to the development of complex higher cortical functions. Being in touch with reality may be considered the most important aspect of human existence. It may range from efforts made for mere indulgence to that of survival. The brain is the control center of all activities, preserving the functional state of the body in relation to the world outside. Most of our engagements with the real world are automatic, but many interactions require voluntary initiation from the brain. In the normal course of development, the brain must cultivate the ability to learn the skills required for defining purposes, setting goals, making action plans, executing them, etc.

Neuropsychological Rehabilitation-Principles and Applications.
DOI: http://dx.doi.org/10.1016/B978-0-12-416046-0.00002-X

The brain must further acquire the ability to initiate and execute actions voluntarily, learn to anticipate [1] the outcome of actions, and monitor both the anticipated and the actual outcome of such actions. Finally, there is a need to learn to change action plans and goals if required, and execute the changed strategies. Cognitive controls help to modulate and support the sensory and motor processes and their interactive controls, which are important functional links for establishing contact with reality, and in responding to and navigating in the real-world.

Modality-specific sensory signals registered in the brain are assigned meaning (encoding), creating information, which is stored as memory traces to enable its later retrieval for recognition and other applications. Such retrieval of memory traces takes place automatically, even when minimal matching signals are processed, and the brain predicts the entity (stimulus) as the information model already available (known) within the memory trace [2,3]. Recognition or perception of familiar entities (world) therefore occurs rapidly. On the other hand, if there is no memory trace available matching the registered pattern of the external entity, there is a need to examine the entity in detail to enable development (learning) of a new piece of information, which serves as the internal model for later recognition. Skills can be acquired with or without awareness (implicit and explicit learning). Skills implicitly learned can be deployed in an implicit manner. Several cognitive processes require the individual to hold onto related but independent pieces of information, which may also include action plans for execution with the data. This may be performed mentally with awareness, and the related information is held in the span of attention of the individual. Span of attention is, therefore, a measure of the quantum of information one can hold online, without needing to retrieve it from memory. The process of holding simultaneously several pieces of information for processing and their execution as per an action plan, also held in the span of attention, refers to the working memory property of the brain. One may retrieve relevant information from memory and hold onto it for current processing as long as required. Such online processing is an important phase of complex motor programming, which raises human behavior above automated conditioned responses to the environment. This may often require one to anticipate the consequence of planned actions as well as monitor the online effects of actions executed [1].

Last but not of the least importance is the ability to learn to experience and express emotions appropriately and relevantly in the social context. Capacity to be emotionally aroused is a vital need for producing the necessary drive required for learning and performing with optimum efficiency. Learning to detect the effects and meaning of emotions in the behavior and speech of others is as important as learning to use emotional affect in one's own speech and behavior. Using emotion as a positive motivation or drive is different from experiencing and expressing negative emotions of anger, fear, aggression, and depression. Emotional experiences are important prerequisites in social interactions, which form an important route for establishing reality contacts. Experiences serve as the only subjective means for establishing contact with reality, and they help to carry out reality verification, despite the fact that experiential interpretations are subjective, as they cannot be objectively shared with others.

# Neuroplasticity and Neurogenesis

There is overwhelming evidence of neuroplasticity and neurogenesis within the brain which supports efforts to retrain and restore cognitive functions even after they are impaired. Plastic adaptation of neurons for reorganization of functions has been demonstrated in the somatosensory, primary visual, and primary auditory cortices, amygdala, hippocampus, and thalamus [4,5], and the effects of neuroplasticity have been supported through several case studies of cognitive retraining as part of neuropsychological rehabilitation programs in brain-injured patients. Development of skills and functional properties in the cognitive domain occurs through the establishment of connectivity among neurons in the brain. According to Hebbian learning theory [6], neurons that fire together get connected and develop cognitive and other functional systems [7–9]. Looking at the architecture of the brain from outside to inside, pathways from sensory receptors reach endpoints in the brain, where processing of the neural signals take place. Multiple functional localizations in the brain occur as a natural outcome of the distribution of the modality-specific sensory inputs. In the same manner, the limbs of the body are controlled in a one-to-one manner in the brain, supporting highly specialized and localized controls for their movements. The capacity of a neuron to become part of a functional neural network is established when it becomes part of the network through connectivity with the other neurons engaged in the same function. Such interconnected neurons form the structural basis for building functional properties in the brain. This property of the neurons supports the concept of neuroplasticity in the brain, and experiences and training can indeed change the functional properties of the neurons. Neuroplasticity refers to the structural changes that various brain cells go through during normal brain development and learning, stressful experiences [10], and as compensatory changes [6]. Acquired brain functions may be lost because of damage and consequent loss of brain cells. This can be compensated partly or fully by restoration of the functions by training new brain cells, and it is considered an important feature of neuroplasticity of the brain cells. Cognitive retraining facilitates participation of greater numbers of neurons in weak functional networks, which result in the restoration of the function fully or partially. In addition to the fact that changes can take place throughout the lifespan, there are also age-related specific functional developments taking place in the brain. Primary acquisition of language ability is a clear example of such age-specific development.

The brain acquires its complex and dynamic functional systems deployed in the monitoring and interpretation of reality through complex interactions, which become varied experiences acquired in life. During acquisition of new functions, abilities, and skills, as part of developmental process, the newly born silent neurons are selected to networks that support the different functions. Structural changes take place at synaptic connections and increased numbers of synaptic connections indicate inclusion of greater numbers of neurons in a functional network. This takes place through normal experiences acquired through skill training, conceptualizations of new ideas and relationships, and mental problem solving, which everyone goes through during the developmental stages. Aging or physical maturation of a person does not stop or retard the capacity of neurons to relearn, alter, and enhance existing abilities. It is now accepted with greater conviction that the behavior of the individual and the experiences that one acquires in the environment can alter neurogenesis of the brain [11]. Evidence exists to indicate that certain areas in the brain can generate neurons throughout life, supporting the presence of continuous neurogenesis [12,13]. New functions can thus be acquired through training if the neurons are available for participation in new functional networks. The abilities and skills learned during the early developmental years are fortified and enriched over years of application. However, learning very new skills at later ages may have impediments for their acquisition and enrichment, especially if it depends on multiple levels of acquisition. Restoration of functions lost because of damage to brain cells requires reexperiencing through retraining. This facilitates the involvement of silent neurons, hitherto not part of any functional network, or neurons designated for other functions may acquire the lost functions, resulting in the process of restoration of the functional status.

Clinical neuropsychological assessment is carried out to determine diffused and/or focal deficits in mode-specific and processing-specific cognitive functioning in patients with brain lesions or trauma, using a battery of specially devised tests. The battery must consist of tests for measuring the diverse and subtle aspects of cognitive processing abilities. The tests use standardized procedures for administration so that they help to reveal the specific deficits in various cognitive and psychomotor functions, which may in turn impair personality and behavior. The deficits may often be part of personality and behavior, which can only be identified as present or not, and tested clinically and not by standardized tests. It is important to have a good idea of the premorbid functioning level of the patient tested in order to determine the nature and the degree of individuals' specific impairment. Premorbid personality and adjustment patterns can be derived with a certain level of reliability by interviewing informants and the patient as well as by making objective assessments of the performance and achievement history of a patient. Similarly, scholastic achievements and verbal skills are also considered indicators of the premorbid intellectual efficiency of a patient. However, there may often be presumptions, and these may pose controversies when used for stringent judgments about a patient's disability. Cognitive retraining must be incorporated as an essential follow-up procedure in clinical examination and treatment before decisions are to be made for rehabilitation of the patient, if necessary. This could address problems related to restoration of neurocognitive functions and the resulting cognitive disability in the patient. The disability obstructs the patient's return to premorbid levels of functioning, making it mandatory to initiate a rehabilitative procedure for the affected individual. A clinical neuropsychological assessment, in this sense, is important for determining the impairment profile of a patient. The most important aspect of a test outcome is the inference of impairments present and their effects on continuing with the premorbid lifestyle and activities of a patient.

# Neuropsychological Impairment in Traumatic Brain Injury in Asian Countries

The epidemiology of traumatic brain injury (TBI) is rather high in India and other Asian countries [14–20]. It is reported that 1.5–2 million persons are injured and about 1 million people die due to head injury. Of these, about 60% have TBI and 20%–25% have falls [15]. Some 15–20% of TBI patients were reported to be under the influence of alcohol at the time of the injury. The condition of a patient after TBI or neurological disease is an important factor in the need for and success of rehabilitation programs. Cognitive, intellectual, emotional, and behavioral problems that may result from brain trauma are considered the major long-term ill effects of TBI for which the patients may require focused help. Factors that influence a patient's selection for cognitive and behavioral retraining in the initial stages are considerations of (a) alertness and attentiveness, (b) level of communication, (c) psychomotor abilities, and (d) emotional stability of the patient. A severely brain-damaged patient may have acute problems in all these four areas. Improvement in the status of impaired cognitive function may take place in a stepwise manner or continuously after a severe brain trauma for a period of 6–16 months. Carrion and Murga [21] found that spontaneous or natural recovery ceases to take place in a sample of severe TBI patients by about 8 months. On a simple reaction time measure, high school athletes were found to take as many as 21 days to return to normality after concussive head injury [22]. Neuropsychological deficits were found to persist even after 1 year of TBI when the injured patients were not provided with any cognitive retraining program [23]. A review of rehabilitation studies [24] showed that cognitive rehabilitation was successful in 78.7% of the 1801 patients with TBI or stroke who were provided such remedial help. The review further supports that cognitive rehabilitation is a logical and imperative follow-up action that must be provided to all patients with brain damage. However, neuropsychological rehabilitation surpasses the boundaries of medical and physical treatments as it engages the family of the patient and the institution, which control occupational participation, and finally social commitments for occupational and social replacements, whenever necessary. It is important to note that cognitive impairment may lead to disabilities in a patient, which can become a handicap for a patient in returning to normal living and working patterns. Cognitive retraining is for restoration of an impaired function or for training patients to learn to achieve the same or close enough results of cognitive problem solving using alternate methods.

# Cognitive Retraining for Restoring Brain Function

Restoration of impaired cognitive functions either fully or partially, with or without compensatory strategies, can be achieved through cognitive retraining programs in patients with most neurological disorders. Cognitive retraining may also help patients in the early stages of neurodegenerative diseases [25]. Any retraining program must provide opportunities for experiencing cognitive challenges, during which the patient's brain learns to generate and test solutions and thereby strengthens the impaired cognitive strategies. Cognitive retraining is recommended when these patients have (a) attention impairment, (b) working memory deficits, (c) impaired executive functions, (d) speech and language disorders, (e) visual field defects and neglects, and (f) loss of cognitive control of behavior and emotions. Rehabilitation of patients with severe brain injuries poses complex problems which are generally absent in the cases of mild to moderate brain injuries. Rehabilitation of degenerative disorders requires differential inputs depending on the magnitude and nature of the functions affected or dysfunctions present at different stages. The disorder may also have legal and epidemiological implications that need to be addressed during the initial neuropsychological assessment and evaluation of the effects of dysfunctions in the lifestyle of the patient.

It is important to differentiate retraining in basic cognitive processing from retraining in specific skills. Attention, working memory, basic visuospatial perception, and encoding may be required for the deployment of all material and mode-specific skills (e.g., reading, writing, arithmetic) and other psychomotor abilities (driving, riding, locomotion). Therefore, retraining in basic processing areas may be viewed differently from retraining in expressive speech and visuospatial abilities required for complex psychomotor skills. Impairment of attention and working memory abilities takes away mental processing capabilities in a person. Alternate methods of expression, in the presence of a handicap, could be taught, and the patient should be trained to make use of and feel comfortable with the new line of expression. This does not mean that the patient may recover all lost memories, unless the loss results from transient global amnesia or the loss has a functional basis that can be repaired psychologically. Despite using a standard retraining technique, each patient adapts to the processing needs presented by the training program in his own idiosyncratic manner and capacity. A therapist can make use of others who live and work with a patient to encourage and facilitate the patient to practice encoding and transcoding the details of those cognitive and expressive activities. Such conceptual enrichment is routinely used as part of brain function therapy (BFT) [26], a computerized cognitive retraining program discussed in detail elsewhere in this chapter. The ability cultivated in the brain by relearning helps one face challenges in life all over again, though the adequacy and success of such attempts may depend on the interplay of several other factors and their effects on the patient. Generally, these factors are not addressed directly in a cognitive retraining program, but they are indeed important considerations for the rehabilitation program and hence need to be addressed by some member of the rehabilitation team. It is useful to monitor the input (training) and output (learned abilities, behavior) variables and their complexities during retraining as it may be worth using those variables or agents which have optimum structural and adaptive properties [27], and the retraining program can then be adjusted according to the assets and liabilities of the patient. Focused cognitive retraining within an institutional setting can easily use programs for retraining of attention, working memory, simple learning, conditioned responses, and response inhibition. However, strengthening higher levels of thinking, learning, and navigational abilities requires handling activities of daily life (ADL) and behavior in special life occasions.

## Effectiveness of Cognitive Retraining

The two basic approaches of retraining programs are direct retraining of the impaired function, which may totally or partially restore the impaired function, and the use of compensatory techniques [28,29], which the person can learn to deploy in place of the impaired ability. There have been several studies in the past decade which have demonstrated the efficacy of computerized cognitive retraining for attention and memory impairment in different types of brain injury/lesion patients [30–35]. Attention retraining was reported to have produced significant improvement in TBI patients [30] and the improved attention enhanced speed and accuracy in recognition tasks in these patients. Retraining using visual scanning techniques was useful for patients who developed unilateral neglect after stroke [36–38]. Gehring et al. [39] have reported facilitatory positive effects of cognitive retraining programs on short-term cognitive complaints and on long-term cognitive performance in the areas of attention and memory in patients in whom tumors of the brain had been surgically removed. Similar confirming and supportive findings have also been reported [40] in the areas of attention and memory. The chief advantages of computerized cognitive retraining are the selection of precision that could be used in the exposure of varied stimuli, precise stepwise changes in inter- and intra-trial intervals, and selection of complexity levels of stimuli and tasks [26,30] used for retraining. The system allows storage of all these details used in each session for later reviewing of the changes in the performance pattern of a patient.

The severity of head injury or damage is an important factor for consideration in planning long-term rehabilitative programs for a patient. This is indeed important for deciding the starting levels of complexities of the tasks [30,41] using computerized retraining methods. Brain damage and its detrimental effects on cognitive and other adaptive functions of the brain have a certain degree of heterogeneity, depending on premorbid pattern and levels of development of the function in the individual. This makes it necessary to make appropriate adaptation of the training program in each patient, if found necessary. It is generally supported [42] that cognitive retraining programs are usually successful in most cases, as they often allow full restoration of the impaired functions. However, such retraining can be successfully carried out only when a program is designed and implemented around a rational processing model. Such processing models can be derived only from already established findings on neurocognitive processing in the brain.

## The BFT Program Modules

BFT is a computer-based program developed by Mukundan [43] in the Clinical Neuropsychology Unit of the National Institute of Mental Health and Neuro Sciences,

Bangalore, with the help of Axxonet System Technologies, between 1995 and 1997. It was developed to provide computerized cognitive retraining program for patients with TBI, other brain lesions, and diseases of the brain. The cases were examined by the author in the Clinical Neuropsychology Unit of NIMHANS during 1996–2003. The BFT program has nine major functional modules, which are presented in the following:

1. *Attention retraining using number and alphabet presentations*: One to four digits or letters are presented on the computer monitor in preset sizes and durations. The patient is instructed to respond to the numbers or letters by calling them out, typing them using the keyboard, or pointing to the same numbers on a chart. The stimuli are exposed for a preset duration or until the subject responds to them. The numbers or letters are presented from a data file prepared by the examiner with preset exposure time. The exposure time of each presentation is generally decreased by 10–50 ms in each session. The program automatically saves the exposure time, responses, and the response time (when keyboard is used) for each presentation.

2. *Attention retraining using word detection*: Three- or four-letter words are presented one after the other on a computer monitor. Both size and exposure duration of the word and inter-trial intervals change according to preset values. The patient is instructed to observe the target word and identify it in either a direct comparison or recall and identify the word from an array of four words presented later. The font used in the target word is different from the fonts of the words in the array to prevent easy visual comparison. A list of words is presented on the monitor from a previously prepared stimulus data file in a random order. Exposure time, inter-trial intervals, and response time are saved by the program.

3. *Speed of reading*: Words or sentences from a data file are presented and horizontally scrolled. The speed of scrolling can be adjusted at the rate of one letter in 100 ms across 10 cm horizontally or at slower rates in a stepwise manner. The subject is instructed to read out the words or continuous text. The speed of scrolling is saved for each presentation. The subject is instructed to read and recall the text immediately or after a delay.

4. *Visuospatial recognition*: The patient is instructed to observe carefully a target figure and identify it from an array of four figures. The comparison figures are presented in equal, smaller, or larger sizes than the target. The identification must be done in direct comparison or from memory. The exposure time of the target and the intra- and inter-trial intervals can be varied, and the actual values are saved by the program along with the response choices of the subject.

5. *Working memory*: The task for the patient is to identify single- or two-digit target numbers and the numbers immediately preceding and following it from a matrix of eight numbers in direct comparisons or from memory, with varying intra-trial intervals. The exposure duration of the target numbers is decreased and the intra-trial interval is increased across sessions, and the details are saved along with the responses chosen by a subject.

6. *Continuous performance*: This is a typical *n*-back test using figures with varying patterns. The patient must respond to repetition of a figure. The rate of change of the figures and exposure duration of each figure can be varied as well as saved by the program.

7. *Temporal sequencing*: The program presents three single-digit numbers one after the other using preset exposure time and intra-trial intervals. After a preset interval, two other numbers are presented one after the other. The patient must report if the last two numbers are in the same sequence as two of the three preceding numbers presented first. The numbers are presented from a stimulus data file. The rate of change of the numbers and exposure duration of each number can be varied, and the responses are saved by the program.

8. *Alphanumeric sequencing*: The patient must learn to recall three to six target digits (numbers or letters) presented on the monitor and, after a preset interval, arrange them by choosing them from an array of numbers or letters presented on another screen. The subject must arrange the numbers in ascending or descending order by selecting each from an array of numbers or letters.

9. *Response inhibition*: This uses a program with a "Go–No-Go" paradigm, which helps the patient learn to inhibit impulsive and forced responses and learn to delay responding as well as choose a response according to a response strategy rather than by habit. The program stores details of all right and wrong responses, including response time and intra-trial intervals used.

Execution of the tasks is carried out at four levels, with the final one requiring the subject to learn to suppress a forced choice and voluntarily select the choice. Level 1 trains the client to learn to make a response to a stimulus figure that appears either at the bottom left or right corner of the screen after the appearance of a central target figure. The subject learns to respond to the matching stimulus with a left- or right-hand finger based on the side on which the stimulus has appeared. In level 2, the stimulus figure randomly differs from the target figure, and the subject must not respond when they do not match. At level 3, the subject is instructed to give a response with the finger of the opposite hand when the target and the stimulus match. At level 4, after the target presentation, two stimuli appear, one in the left and the other in the right bottom corners, one after the other. The subject learns to make a response only when the second stimulus matches the first and the target, but the response is made after the appearance of the second stimulus by the finger matching the side where the first stimulus appeared.

# Findings with BFT-Based Cognitive Retraining

The results of retraining efforts using BFT are in line with those of other computer-aided cognitive programs discussed in this chapter. Use of the computer for cognitive retraining facilitates presentation of a variety of stimuli and cognitive tasks with gradually increasing difficulty levels across sessions. Difficulty level of a task can be controlled not only by varying its complexity but also by reducing exposure time and other features of visual presentations. However, it is important that each task should allow deployment of a neuropsychological–cognitive principle, which is strengthened in the patient across repeated retraining trials. Use of a computer is only for a controlled presentation of the cognitive tasks. Some of the findings obtained using BFT program are discussed here.

## Retraining for Restoration of Attention

Three attention-related abilities generally impaired in TBI and other lesions affecting the frontal lobes are (1) absence of spontaneous arousal of attention when a new stimulus appears in the personal environment of the patient, (2) inability to selectively or intentionally focus attention on a stimulus or object, person, or entity in the personal environment, and (3) absence of habituation of arousal of attention to irrelevant stimuli [44,23,45]. Retraining of attention using computer-based tasks and the deployment of skills of attention in real-life situations may have marked differences. For moving around a building, walking or driving, the person must acquire the ability to attend selectively as well as ignore irrelevant stimuli. Impairment of such ability can result in a person encountering life-threatening situations. Hence, there is natural caution as well as fear of consequences, if a person does not adequately apply attention to his daily life situations. One learns to deploy them habitually from early childhood experiences of ADL. Computerized retraining of attention does not offer such reality contacts, though performance is judged in terms of successes and errors in each retraining trial. This indeed allows immense freedom and strength for the use of the program despite repeated failures. It is a common finding during BFT training in patients with severe brain injury that many of them require a single-digit number or letter to be presented for several seconds on the monitor before they recognize and produce a response to it. Thorough retraining sessions conducted every day for about 15 min for 2 weeks on this module alone; the exposure time required for recognition reduces to a few hundred (600–1000 ms) milliseconds for four-digit numbers or letters. By the end of a month, they may correctly recognize the four numbers or letters presented for about 200 ms (Figure 2.1). Concurrently, arousal of attention to irrelevant stimuli is also gradually attenuated, as seen in attention-deficit hyperactivity disorder (ADHD) children, who undergo attention retraining along with retraining in response inhibition. The patient is encouraged and helped in the initial stages for learning to work on the test by the therapist. The patient is provided with opportunities to give responses by directly responding on the keyboard, pointing to printed numbers and letters, or orally responding, according to the preference and capability of each patient. The therapist and other members of the family can also supervise ADL in which attentional skills are to be applied with caution. The

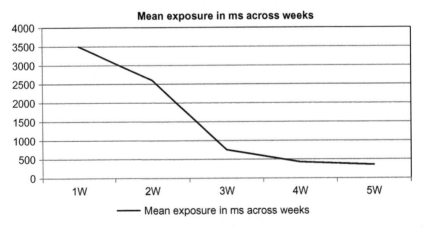

**Figure 2.1 Attention retraining across weeks 1–5 using BFT.** Exposure duration required for recognition falls from mean 3500 to 370 ms over the fifth week during retraining in TBI patients (sample = 32).

capacity for attentional skills in ADL is restored slowly, though it may not exactly coincide with the marked improvements seen in computer-based training programs, in the early stages. If the attention training in the ADL does not reach the necessary safe levels, despite significant improvement seen in the computer-based training programs, the patient must be advised to avoid risky situations in the ADL.

The modules of Word Recognition and Reading Speed Enhancement also provide retraining in the domain of attention. The exposure time of the target words and the speed of flow of the text used for reading on the screen are gradually changed across sessions for increasing difficulty levels, and the subject is gradually trained to read out faster. He is further encouraged to recall the contents of the text used in each session immediately and at the end of the training program. Both TBI and other lesion patients with moderate to severe injury or dysfunction invariably have difficulty in quick recognition of the words, and the module gradually helps in improving focused attention and recognition. The two modules used one after the other help to establish familiarity and quick recognition of large numbers of words and reduce distractibility.

## Retraining of Working Memory

Working memory is another important area suitable for computerized retraining programs. Significant working memory improvement has been reported in ADHD children using such programs [46]. Working memory retraining is a significant part of the BFT program. The programs enable recognition of numbers and words, allowing the patient to hold onto the numbers or words for increasing durations and then use them for further processing in a sequential manner. BFT modules allow the retraining of the two components of working memory, namely (a) the central executive and (b) the buffer memory [2,47–49]. They allow retraining of the three central executive components of (1) holding onto plan(s) of action, (2) execution of the plan(s) of action sequentially, which may include set shifting, and (3) deploying the necessary skills for execution of the plans of action. The other component of the working memory is the use of buffer memory for holding onto the retrieved, externally presented, as well as computed data in verbal and/or visual modes. The buffer must also hold onto the results processed through sequential and/or deductive processing. Simple examples for working memory could be a simple deduction of series of number from 1 to 20, or repeated serial subtraction of 4 to 40. The working memory test, initially called the delayed response ability test, is part of the NIMHANS neuropsychological battery [44,23], and it is a very sensitive test for frontal dysfunction. Retraining in working memory processing, therefore, is of paramount importance in any head injury or lesion patient as it rekindles the mental problem-solving abilities in the affected individual. Even if the person is handicapped in some sensorimotor functions, ability to process information mentally using working memory is an extraordinary talent, which allows one to contribute meaningfully in life.

The BFT program module for working memory starts with simple tasks in which the patient must observe and then hold onto single- or two-digit numbers and search out numbers greater and lesser than by 1 in a matrix of numbers presented on the screen. The patient must either key in those numbers or call them out by pointing at them one after the other. The next level task consists of arranging numbers or letters [2–6] displayed on the monitor for a preset exposure time, in ascending or descending order, by choosing them by the mouse from a randomly presented matrix of numbers or letters on another screen after a preset delay. The ability to hold onto four digits of numbers or letters and then to arrange them mentally in ascending or descending order indicates near-normalization of the working memory function in the training situation. The spatial comparison test offers working memory functions in addition to spatial analysis and synthesis. The word recognition test also has a working memory component, as the subject is required to hold onto a word and use the mental image for its identification from an array of words, which appears on the screen after a certain interval. Daily training for a duration of 15–30 min in two sessions is found to improve the working memory ability in patients within 20–25 days. However, the type of processing and material specificity used by each individual varies and hence a general-purpose working memory retraining may only partially help a patient in occupational rehabilitation in the early stage of recovery.

Overall improvement in working memory functions may be clinically apparent over a period of 3–4 weeks of retraining, though the level may still not reach the inferred premorbid levels in all patients. Since the accuracy and speed factors of working memory ability are functions of the complexity levels of the tasks used, it may be difficult to either predict or make a decisive judgment about the recovery status. It is easier to find significant improvement on computer-based working memory tests than in ADL. Patients may learn a task in the job situation requiring working memory engagement more convincingly than a complex computer-based working memory task. However, the most important aspect of the retraining program is the opportunity to relearn the basic cognitive process in a systematic and stepwise manner with increasing levels of difficulty, which facilitates the restoration of the impaired complex function.

### Visuospatial Analysis and Synthesis

Examination of visual space and its analysis for the purpose of recognition of spatial attributes is an important domain for cognitive retraining of patients who have significant right-hemisphere damage or dysfunction. Visuospatial analysis and visual integration are important cognitive abilities required to differentiate and recognize visuospatial attributes of objects and to use the visual space in which one lives and works. Such visual-perceptual errors are different from a total failure of visual recognition identified as visual agnosia. Visual-perceptual and integrative failures are easily detected in neuropsychological performance tests, namely, block design test, object assembly test, Alexander's pass-along test, complex figure test, Bender Gestalt test, and other visuospatial drawing and construction tests. Loss or impairment in visuospatial functions can cause difficulties for the individual in spatial orientation in movements, impairments in spatial coordination, perceptual assessment of relative size of objects, spatial distances and positions, and other spatial attributes, all of which can disturb sensorimotor contacts with reality.

Retraining in visuospatial perception and coordination can be easily carried out by the use of computerized programs. However, it may not be appropriate to presume that retraining in the two-dimensional video-space of the computer screen will automatically help restore the lost functional capabilities, especially those related to psychomotor handling of real personal space. The BFT has programs which help to distinguish differences in size and patterns using direct comparison and working memory paradigms. Visual-perceptual impairments generally occur in TBI cases as well as lesions of occipital–parietal–temporal lobes. Retraining using exposure time of the target patterns for long to very short durations helps the individual learn to differentiate and recognize patterns in a rapid manner. Tests of visual perception incorporating pattern construction and drawing are important ingredients of any neuropsychological battery of tests. The BFT program allows perceptual discrimination based on size and pattern complexity. Right frontal and temporal lesions have adverse effects on visual-perceptual drawing and construction tests as visual integrative ability can be impaired by lesions [44,45] in these areas other than the direct effects seen because of posterior and right-hemisphere lesions. Visual-perceptual understanding can be learned using direct spatial comparison of target figures with choices and in the continuous performance modules of the BFT, whereas memory-based comparisons of the target figures may require one to hold onto visual images or recreate them and verbally transcode the visual target figures. This has been demonstrated in the visual learning and memory function tests of the NIMHANS neuropsychological battery. Visual learning is found to be impaired even in patients with left frontal and temporal lesions, which is explained by the impairment in verbal transcoding skills shown by patients of left anterior and medial (frontal and temporal) lesions [3]. However, visual-perceptual deficits shown by the left-lesion patients significantly differ from the deficits shown by right-lesion patients. Right lesions produce spatial distortions and macro- and micrographia, whereas fragmentation and missing features of the visual figure are seen in left lesions. This is evident in the first three trials and in the delayed recall trial of the test. On the other hand, the fourth trial, in which the subject is instructed to copy the design, typical left-lesion deficits described above are infrequent or absent, unless drawing is impaired by the presence of construction apraxia.

## Response Inhibition Ability

Response to a stimulus could be a learned conditioned response and it might serve an important purpose in the domain of social conditioning of the individual. However, there are situations when individuals must make a choice and decide the course of action (i.e., intentional or voluntary actions) instead of responding in a conditioned manner. Ability to inhibit conditioned responses is therefore an important component of complex motor programming required for executive functions, especially related to navigational activities, in which each individual has to participate. Response inhibition ability refers to the cognitive ability to inhibit a conditioned response, and initiate and execute an alternate response/action as per a strategic plan. The BFT program helps patients relearn the ability to (a) inhibit irrelevant responses and (b) delay relevant responses so they learn to make them at appropriate point in time.

The anterior cingulate cortex (ACC) has a significant role in exercising cognitive controls in stimulus–response selection and execution, and these have been indicated in clinical lesion and neuroimaging studies [50]. Neuroimaging evidence has been elicited showing the role of the ACC in mediating response competition and conflicts [51–53], online input monitoring [54], selective attention [55], and divided attention [56]. These are some of the executive controls exercised by the prefrontal cortex which may be impaired in TBI and other diseases/lesions affecting the prefrontal cortex. Such executive controls are characteristics of the complex motor programming system, which the individual engages for navigational self-controls in the execution of all goal-directed activities. Loss of ability for selective attention or inadequate development of the ability results in poor habituation of attentional arousal to irrelevant stimuli and consequent distractibility. The response inhibition ability is, therefore, required for inhibition or delay of responses and for enabling response selection based on selective effects as desired or planned by the individual. Impairment of this ability is seen in varying degrees in various frontal lobe dysfunctions occurring in TBI and other lesions affecting the frontal lobes. It is also seen in the early developmental stages in children prior to the development of frontal autonomy. ADHD seen in children is a common condition seen with this debility, as response inhibition ability does not develop adequately. Retraining in attentional selection and response inhibition plays very important roles in attaining mastery over responses and actions.

TBI patients, patients with frontal lobe dysfunction, and children with ADHD who respond well to such training programs take 3–4 weeks before they learn to reach the fourth level and make about 50% correct responses. Frontal patients have a conspicuously significant tendency to choose a response opposite to what is actually prompted. ADHD children learn this with practice and show marked improvement in their behavioral responses as it results in reduction of distractibility and irrelevant responsiveness. Significant effects might be seen in their scholastic performance when performance is compared to their pretraining levels. Significant improvements in behavior and performance on neuropsychological tests have been found to occur with a cognitive retraining of 3–4 weeks in TBI patients with moderate severity. The improvement is often considered complete by the patients when the severity of TBI is minimal. Within 2 weeks of continuous retraining, many of these patients prefer to start training in real work situations rather than visit the clinic for specialized retraining. Clinical and neuropsychological recovery patterns were studied [23] in TBI patients who did not have the benefit of cognitive retraining or any specialized rehabilitative help (as such help was not available) after sustaining the head injury. Forty-two TBI patients (40 male, 2 female) with a mean age of 33.2 years (SD = 11.2) were assessed on neuropsychological 3, 6, and 12 months after the initial admission, and their performance was compared with that of a normal control group ($n = 26$) matched for age and education. On the Glasgow Comma Scale [57], 24 patients had scores in the 6–8 range, 16 had scores in the 9–11 range, and 2 had scores of 4 and 5 during admission immediately after sustaining the injury. Maximum rate of clinical recovery was seen in the patient group in the assessment 1 month after the trauma. Approximately 76% of the patients were neurologically normal at first

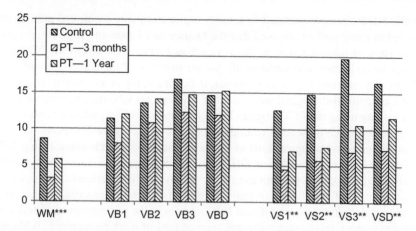

**Figure 2.2  Mean scores on the working memory test,** the four trials of verbal (VB1, VB2, VB3, VBD) and visual (VS1, VS2, VS3, VSD) learning and memory functions tests of the control group ($n = 26$) and of the TBI patients in their third month and 1-year assessments, who were not provided with any cognitive retraining program [23]. Significance of mean difference ***$P < 0.001$, **$P < 0.01$.

month and 83% were found to be neurologically normal during the third month assessment. Neuropsychological assessment was carried out by the tests that were being validated using CT scan and neurosurgical findings (NIMHANS neuropsychological battery, [44]). The initial neuropsychological assessment was conducted a month after the trauma. The mean scores of performance of patients on tests of working memory and verbal and visual learning memory functions are shown in the third month and 1-year assessments in comparison with the control group in Figure 2.2. These tests showed significant impairment in the areas of visual scanning, visuospatial organization, working memory, visual integration, visual learning, and visual memory in the third month of assessment. The repeat trials of the complex figure and passages provide information about learning/encoding over trials. In the third month assessment, the patient group did not show significant impairment on ideational fluency and verbal learning and memory function tests (Figure 2.2) compared to the control group. However, they had significant impairment on the working memory test as well as on the immediate and delayed recalls of the visual learning and memory functions test in their third month and 1-year comparisons (Figure 2.2) with the control group, despite the fact the mean scores of the patient group did show improvement over the 1 year. A majority of the patients (69%) continued having difficulties in social adjustment and had emotional problems even 1 year after the trauma. It was explained in the light of a contemporary hypothesis [58] that the right-hemisphere functions developmentally take shape as well as recover at significantly slower rates than the left-hemisphere functions when they are impaired.

A subgroup of the above patients underwent an evoked and event-related potential study [59] to determine their attentional recovery pattern. Twenty-six patients were assessed for eliciting attentional components in visual and auditory modes.

The P1–N1–P2 complex related to sensory registration and attentional arousal [60] recorded in these patients showed that the latency of P1 (sensory registration) component showed normalization in the 1-month assessment. However, the N1 (attentional arousal) latency was significantly greater than that of the normal control group in the third month and 1-year assessments, indicating delay in attentional arousal.

Repeat neuropsychological assessment of TBI patients who have undergone cognitive retraining using the BFT program has shown statistically significant improvement [30] in performance on several neuropsychological tests. Figure 2.3 shows the mean scores on neuropsychological tests in pre- and postcognitive retraining (using BFT) assessments in a group ($n=25$) of TBI, tumor, or stroke patients. Cognitive retraining was provided for periods ranging from 20 to 45 days to these patients. The postcognitive retraining profile indicates overall change in the cognitive processing capacity of the individual. Statistically significant improvement in the postretraining performance compared to pretraining assessment was seen on tests of working memory (WM), visual (VS), and verbal (VB) learning and memory functions (Figure 2.3). Significant improvement was noticed on the immediate and delayed recalls of the repeat trials of verbal and visual tests. Comparison of posttraining neuropsychological assessment mean scores of the TBI patients with normative data did not show any significant difference in the above tests, though the patient group had lower mean scores than the normative data on the trial making, object assembly, and block design tests. Interestingly, visual and auditory N1 latencies were normalized (compared to the normative data of the laboratory) in this group of patients (visual N1 = 148 ms, auditory N1 = 106 ms) in their posttraining assessments. This was significantly different from the earlier findings on the TBI patients who did not receive cognitive retraining and

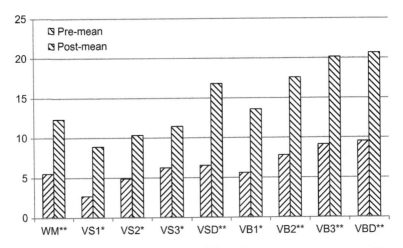

**Figure 2.3 Mean scores of pre- and postcognitive retraining assessments in working memory (WM),** the three immediate recall trials (VS1, VS2, VS3 and VB1, VB2, VB3), and the delayed recall trials (VSD and VBD) of visual and verbal learning memory functions tests [30] in 25 TBI, tumor, or stroke patients who were trained by the BFT program. Significance levels for within group pre- and postcomparisons: $*P < 0.01$, $**P < 0.001$.

continued to have significantly delayed latency even at the 1-year assessment. The improvements seen in the neuropsychological tests support the positive facilitating effects of the cognitive retraining in the patients who suffered from TBI.

Restoration of cognitive functions using retraining programs does not necessarily mean that the patients regain total cognitive controls over their behavior and emotions in daily activities of life (DAL). Behavioral modification techniques and counseling may be required by some of the patients for achieving this control. There is need to enrich the cognitive advantage by behavioral supports, and this forms an important aspect of total rehabilitation of a brain-damaged patients. The cognitive enrichment of behavior must be planned and designed for each patient and it must be carefully monitored [26,32]. Computer-controlled cognitive retraining has the immense advantage of control of presentation of the stimuli and seeking a variety of response patterns. Difficulty levels can be easily adjusted and made suitable for each patient in terms of exposure durations, inter- and intra-trial intervals, and the complexity of the cognitive problem-solving tasks. We could not have achieved those controls manually if the retraining tasks were administered without computer aid. With BFT, it has been the practice that the difficulty levels are adjusted such that the patient can correctly respond to between 50% and 70% or more trials in each session. The difficulty level is minimally increased in each session, allowing the patient to learn to cope with each presentation with immense self-confidence. Further, this provides the therapist with the opportunity to help the patient deal with the difficulties in a systematic manner by adjusting the requirements of DAL. For example, a patient who has difficulty carrying out a simple mental arithmetic problem is allowed to practice it first in writing and learn the strategy or steps and then gradually learn to carry it out mentally. A patient may learn to carry out mental shopping and calculate the total amount he has to pay after purchasing several items. Once the patient has learned to carry out a simple task correctly, the difficulty level is gradually increased, and the patient is provided with feedback about his improvement. However, training in complex psychomotor activities such as playing a ball game or driving cannot be practiced with the BFT program, though there are other computer programs which may help even in those efforts.

## Conclusions

All societies consider a head trauma accidently acquired to be unfortunate, as it often occurs because of avoidable human errors, unlike other diseases, which may occur because of unpredicted and unavoidable reasons, despite efforts to avoid being subjected to them. Social opportunities and privileges available for treatment and rehabilitation differ across societies and countries. However, scientific understanding can be made available for all in a uniform manner. The fact that impaired cognitive functions can often be successfully restored is convincing proof of neuroplasticity and neurogenesis of the brain. Agewise decline in cognitive abilities or "mild cognitive impairment" [61,62] has become a controversial issue. There is increasing agreement that applying such diagnostic classifications in a general sense to geriatric population is erroneous, despite the fact that "aging-associated cognitive decline

(AACD)" is mentioned by the American Psychiatric Association (1993) and ICD-10 of the World Health Organization (1993) as a natural process. Age-associated normal cognitive decline is an experience of many aging persons, though the scientific etiology is not yet clear. The whole issue is often considered controversial [63], requiring further verification. It is reported that old and young-old [64, 65] persons indeed experience such decline. However, they may also have reduced cognitive engagement in those areas where they report such cognitive decline, especially memory-related deficits. Natural decline in the skeleto-muscular system and the consequent changes in lifestyle cause withdrawal from cognitive and intellectual challenges in many individuals in their active occupational and professional domains. This may lead to decline in mental processing, especially working memory–related problems in their occupations, causing withdrawal from large knowledge databanks which the person would have otherwise used on a daily basis. Temporary loss of memory or difficulty in retrieval of information from such data domains may be the consequent effect in the affected individual. This may be wrongly labeled as a natural decline of cognitive abilities. The fact that there are many who do remain cognitively active and do not have such declines is an important factor for consideration. It is understood and accepted that there may be changes in the quality and degree of cognitive challenges and stimulations sought out and experienced by the aged as well as youth. The cognitive demands and information realms may change significantly, and individuals may have difficulty recalling from areas that have become redundant and seldom probed into. This would not be considered a true decline as such a decline in memory may be a normal phenomenon that can be restored if one reengages and carries out cognitive exercises in those areas. This is a frequently encountered situation with all individuals and more often in aged persons. On the other hand, decline in autobiographic memory may have a significant clinical diagnostic implication, and one must take considerable care to rule out that the cognitive declines seen are not the early signs of a degenerative or deficiency disorder.

Computerized cognitive retraining programs have provided excellent methods for both restoration and enhancement of cognitive functions in patients and individuals of all age groups. Computer-aided presentation of cognitive tasks helps in the systematic enhancement of speed and accuracy measures as well as complexity of the tasks. These cognitive exercises have become the most effective choice, not only for restoration of cognitive impairment in brain trauma but also for alleviating the discomfort and disadvantages experienced by those in early dementia as well as for those with cognitive decline resulting from the absence of higher levels of cognitive practices in everyday life.

# References

[1] Sperry, R. W. (1950). Neural basis of the spontaneous optokinetic response produced visual inversion. *Journal of Comparative and Physiological Psychology, 43*(6), 482–489.
[2] Biederman, I. (1987). Recognition-by-components: A theory of human image understanding. *Psychological Review, 94*, 115–147.

[3] Mukundan, C. R. (2007). *Brain experience: Neuroexperiential perspectives of brain–mind*. New Delhi: Atlantis Publication.

[4] Buonomano, D. V., & Merzenich, M. M. (1998). Cortical plasticity: From synapse to maps. *Annual Review of Neuroscience, 21*, 149–186.

[5] Stiles, J. (2000). Neural plasticity and cognitive development. *Developmental Neuropsychology, 18*(2), 237–272.

[6] Hebb, D. O. (1961). Distinctive features of learning in the higher animal. In J. F. Delafresnaye (Ed.), *Brain mechanisms and learning*. London: Oxford University Press.

[7] Fernando, C., Goldstein, R., & Szathmáry, E. (2010). The neuronal replicator hypothesis. *Neural Computation, 22*(11), 2809–2857.

[8] Simpson, H. D., Mortimer, D., & Goodhill, G. J. (2009). Theoretical models of neural circuit development. *Current Topics in Developmental Biology, 87*, 1–51.

[9] Munakata, Y., & Pfaffly, J. (2004). Hebbian learning and development. *Developmental Science, 7*(2), 141–148.

[10] Butz, M., Wörgötter, F., & van Ooyen, A. (2009). Activity-dependent structural plasticity. *Brain Research Review, 60*(2), 287–305.

[11] Gage, F. H. (2004). Basic research: Structural plasticity of the adult brain. In J. -P. Macher & M. -A. Crocq (Eds.), *Dialogues in clinical neuroscience neuroplasticity* (Vol. 6, pp. 135–142). France: Les Laboratoires Servier. No. 2.

[12] Gage, F. H., Ray, J., & Fisher, L. J. (1995). Isolation, characterization, and use of stem cells from the CNS. *Annual Review of Neuroscience, 18*, 159–192.

[13] Horner, P. J., & Gage, F. H. (2000). Regenerating the damaged central nervous system. *Nature, 407*, 963–970.

[14] Gururaj, G. (2008). Road traffic deaths, injuries and disabilities in India: Current scenario. *The National Medical Journal of India, 21*, 14–20.

[15] Gururaj, G. (2002). Epidemiology of traumatic brain injuries: Indian scenario. *Neurological Research, 24*, 24–28.

[16] Gururaj, G. (1995). An epidemiological approach to prevention—Prehospital care and rehabilitation in neurotrauma. *Neurology India, 43*(3), 95–105.

[17] Aravind, K., Sanjeev, L., Deepak, A., Ravi, R., & Dogra, T. D. (2008). Fatal road traffic accidents and their relationship with head injuries: An epidemiological survey of five years. *Indian Journal of Neurotrauma, 5*(2), 63–67.

[18] Ghaffar, A., Hyder, A. A., & Masud, T. I. (2004). The burden of road traffic injuries in developing countries: The 1st national injury survey of Pakistan. *Public Health, 118*(3), 211–217.

[19] Puvanachandra, P., & Adnan, A. H. (2009). The burden of traumatic brain injury in Asia: A call for research. *Pakistan Journal of Neurological Science, 4*(1), 27–32.

[20] Tabish, A., Lone, N. A., Afzal, W. M., & Salam, A. (2006). The incidence and severity of injury in children hospitalized for traumatic brain injury in Kashmir. *Injury, 37*(5), 410–415.

[21] Carrion, J. L., & Murga, F. M. (2001). Spontaneous recovery of cognitive functions after severe brain injury: When are neurocognitive sequelae established? *Revista Espanola de Neuropsycholiga, 3*(3), 58–67.

[22] Covassin, T., Elbin, R. J., & Nakayama, Y. (2010). Tracking neurocognitive performance following concussion in high school athletes. *The Physician and Sportsmedicine, 38*(4), 87–93.

[23] Mukundan, C. R., Narayana Reddy, G. N., Hegde, A. S., Shankar, J., & Kaliaperumal, V. G. (1987). Neuropsychological and clinical recovery in patients with head trauma. *NIMHANS Journal, 5*(1), 23–31.

[24] Cicerone, K. D., Dahlberg, C., Malec, J. F., Langebahn, D. M., Felicetti, T., Kneipp, S., et al. (2005). Evidence-based cognitive rehabilitation: Updated review of the literature from 1998 through 2002. *Archives of Physical Medicine and Rehabilitation, 86,* 1681–1692.

[25] Fleischman, D. A. (2007). Repetition priming in aging and Alzheimer's disease: An integrative review and future directions. *Cortex, 43*(7), 889–897.

[26] Mukundan, C. R. (2003). Brain function therapy and conceptual enrichment. *Proceedings of the national workshop in clinical neuropsychology.* Bangalore, India: National Institute of Mental Health & Neuro Sciences Publication.

[27] Kulvicius, T., Kolodziejski, C., Tamosiunaite, M., Porr, B., & Wörgötter, F. (2010). Behavioral analysis of differential Hebbian learning in closed-loop systems. *Biological Cybernetics, 103*(4), 255–271.

[28] Backman, L., & Dixon, R. A. (1992). Psychological compensation: A theoretical framework. *Psychological Bulletin, 112,* 259–283.

[29] Vanderploeg, R. D., Collins, R. C., Sigford, B., Date, E., Schwab, K., & Warden, D. (2006). Practical and theoretical considerations in designing rehabilitation trials: The DVBIC cognitive-didactic versus functional-experiential treatment study experience. *The Journal of Head Trauma Rehabilitation, 21,* 179–193.

[30] Shailaja, C., Anita, R., & Mukundan, C. R. (2009). Technology in rehabilitation: A computer based cognitive retraining program for patients with head injury. *Indian Journal of Clinical Psychology, 1*(1), 11–22.

[31] Alessandra, S., Achille, M., Laura, M., Eugenio, P., Marco, F., Gianluigi, M., et al. (2004). Computer-aided retraining of memory and attention in people with multiple sclerosis: A randomized, double-blind controlled trial. *Journal of the Neurological Sciences, 222*(1), 99–104.

[32] Ansel, B. M., & Weinrich, M. (2002). Computerized approaches to communication retraining after stroke. *Current Atherosclerosis, 4*(4), 291–295.

[33] McAllister, T. W., McDonald, B. C., Flashman, L. A., & Saykin, A. J. (2002). Executive dysfunction following traumatic brain injury: Neural substrates and treatment strategies. *NeuroRehabilitation, 17*(4), 333–344.

[34] Palmese, C. A., & Raskin, S. A. (2000). The rehabilitation of attention in individuals with mild traumatic brain injury, using the APT-II programme. *Brain Injury, 14*(6), 535–548.

[35] Sohlberg, M. M., McLaughlin, K. A., Pavese, A., Heidrich, A., & Posner, M. I. (2000). Evaluation of attention process training and brain injury education in persons with acquired brain injury. *Journal of Clinical and Experimental Neuropsychology, 22,* 656–676.

[36] Jutai, J. W., Bhogal, S. K., Foley, N. C., Bayley, M., Teasell, R. W., & Speechley, M. R. (2003). Treatment of visual perceptual disorders post stroke. *Topics in Stroke Rehabilitation, 10*(2), 77–106.

[37] Polanowska, K., Seniów, J., Paprot, E., Le niak, M., & Członkowska, A. (2009). Left-hand somatosensory stimulation combined with visual scanning training in rehabilitation for post-stroke hemi neglect: A randomized, double-blind study. *Neuropsychological Rehabilitation, 19*(3), 364–382.

[38] Luukkainen-Markkula, R., Tarkka, I. M., Pitkänen, K., Sivenius, J., & Hämäläinen, H. (2009). Rehabilitation of hemispatial neglect: A randomized study using either arm activation or visual scanning training. *Restorative Neurology and Neuroscience, 27*(6), 663–672.

[39] Gehring, K., Sitskoorn, M. M., Gundy, C. M., Sikkes, S. A., Klein, M., Postma, T. J., et al. (2009). Cognitive rehabilitation in patients with gliomas: A randomized, controlled trial. *Journal of Clinical Oncology, 27*(22), 3712–3722.

[40] Tsaousides, T., & Gordon, W. A. (2009). Cognitive rehabilitation following traumatic brain injury: Assessment to treatment. *The Mount Sinai Journal of Medicine, 76*(2), 173–181.

[41] Hoskison, M. M., Moore, A. N., Hu, B., Orsi, S., Kobori, N., & Dash, P. K. (2009). Persistent working memory dysfunction following traumatic brain injury: Evidence for a time-dependent mechanism. *Neuroscience, 159*(2), 483–491.

[42] Halligan, P. W., & Wade, D. T. (2005). *Effectiveness of rehabilitation for cognitive deficits*. New York, NY: Oxford University Press.

[43] Mukundan, C. R. (1996). Introduction of brain function therapy: Computer based cognitive retraining program for brain damaged patients: *Proceedings of the national work-shop in Clinical Neuropsychology*. Bangalore, India: National Institute of Mental Health & Neuro Sciences Publication.

[44] Mukundan, C. R., Rao, S. L., Jain, V. K., Jayakumar, P. N., & Shilaja, K. (1991). Neuropsychological assessment: A cross validation study with neuroradiological/operative findings in patients with cerebral hemisphere lesions. *Pharmacopsychoecologia, 4*, 33–39.

[45] Mukundan, C. R. (1996). NIMHANS neuropsychological battery: Test descriptions, instructions, clinical data and interpretation: *Proceedings of the national workshop in Clinical Neuropsychology*. Bangalore, India: National Institute of Mental Health & Neuro Sciences Publication.

[46] Klingberg, T., Fernell, E., Olesen, P. J., Johnson, M., Gustafsson, P., Dahlström, K., et al. (2005). Computerized training of working memory in children with ADHD—A randomized controlled trial. *Journal of American Academy of Child and Adolescent Psychiatry, 44*(2), 177–186.

[47] Jonides, J., Smith, E. E., Koeppe, R. A., Awh, E., Minoshima, S., & Mintun, M. A. (1993). Spatial working memory in humans as revealed by PET. *Nature, 363*, 623–625.

[48] D'Esposito, M., Detre, J. A., Alsop, D. C., Shin, R. K., Atlas, S., & Grossman, M. (1995). The neural basis of the central executive system of working memory. *Nature, 378*, 279–281.

[49] Andres, P. (2003). Frontal cortex as the central executive of working memory: Time to revise our view. *Cortex, 39*, 871–895.

[50] Braver, T. S, Barch, D. M., Gray, J. R., Molfese, D. L., & Snyder, A. (2001). Anterior cingulate cortex and response conflict: Effects of frequency, inhibition and errors. *Cerebral Cortex, 11*(9), 825–836.

[51] Barch, D. M., Braver, T. S., Akbudak, E., Conturo, T., Ollinger, J., & Snyder, A. V. (2001). Anterior cingulate cortex and response conflict: Effects of response modality and processing domain. *Cerebral Cortex, 11*, 837–848.

[52] Botvinick, M. M., Nystrom, L., Fissel, K., Carter, C. S., & Cohen, J. D. (1999). Conflict monitoring versus selection-for action in anterior cingulate cortex. *Nature, 402*, 179–181.

[53] Casey, B. J., Thomas, K. M., Welsh, T. F., Badgaiyan, R., Eccard, C. H., Jennings, J. R., et al. (2000). Dissociation of response conflict, attentional selection, and expectancy with functional magnetic resonance imaging (fMRI). *Proceedings of the National Academy of Sciences, USA, 97*, 8728–8733.

[54] Carter, C. S., Macdonald, A. M., Botvinick, M., Ross, L. L., Stenger, A., Noll, D., et al. (2000). Parsing executive processes: Strategic versus evaluative functions of the anterior cingulate cortex. *Proceedings of the National Academy of Sciences, USA, 97*, 1944–1948.

[55] Kiehl, K. A., Laurens, K. R., Duty, T. L., Forster, B. B., & Liddle, P. F. (2001). Neural sources involved in auditory target detection and novelty processing: An event-related fMRI study. *Psychophysiology, 38,* 133–142.

[56] Corbetta, M., Miezin, F. M., Dobmeyer, S., Shulman, G. L., & Petersen, S. E. (1991). Selective and divided attention during visual discriminations of shape, color, and speed: Functional anatomy by positron emission tomography. *Journal of Neuroscience, 11,* 2383–2402.

[57] Teasdale, G., & Jennett, B. (1974). Assessment of coma and impaired consciousness. A practical scale. *The Lancet, 2*(7872), 81–84.

[58] Weintraub, S., & Measulam, M. M. (1983). Developmental learning disabilities of the right hemisphere: Emotional, interpersonal and cognitive components. *Archives of Neurology, 40,* 463–468.

[59] Mukundan, C. R., Reddy, Narayana, Hegde, A. S., & Shankar, Jayathi (1990). Effects of long term recovery on the middle latency components of evoked potential responses in head injury patients. *Pharmacopsychoecologia, 2,* 49–56.

[60] Mukundan, C. R. (1986). *Evoked Potentials: Basic Principles and Methods.* Bangalore, India: National Institute of Mental Health & Neuro Sciences Publications. No. 11.

[61] Ritchie, K., Artero, S., & Touchon, J. (2001). Classification criteria for mild cognitive impairment: A population-based validation study. *Neurology, 56*(1), 37–42.

[62] Artero, S., Touchon, J., & Ritchie, K. (2001). Disability and mild cognitive impairment: A longitudinal population-based study. *International Journal of Geriatric Psychiatry, 16*(11), 1092–1097.

[63] Salthouse, T. A. (2009). When does-age related cognitive decline begin? *Neurobiology of Aging, 30*(4), 507–514.

[64] Deary, I. J., Corley, J., Gow, A. J., Harris, S. E., Houlihan, L. M., Marioni, R. E., et al. (2009). Age-associated cognitive decline. *British Medical Bulletin, 92*(1), 135–152.

[65] Schönknecht, P., Pantel, J., Kruse, A., & Schroder, J. (2005). Prevalence and natural course of aging-associated cognitive decline in a population-based sample of young–old subjects. *American Journal of Psychiatry, 162,* 2071–2077.

# 3 Neuropsychological Rehabilitation: Healing the Wounded Brain Through a Holistic Approach

## J. Rajeswaran, D. Sadana, H. Kashyap

Clinical Neuropsychology Unit, Department of Clinical Psychology, National Institute of Mental Health and Neurosciences (NIMHANS), Bangalore, Karnataka, India

Neuropsychological rehabilitation starts from the premise that if functions are not completely obliterated, there is a chance that they can be restored through the brain's ability to heal and adapt. It is still unresolved as to what degree the improvement in neuropsychological functions is due to spontaneous recovery or to the neuropsychological rehabilitation techniques used. Neuropsychological rehabilitation is an ongoing process and should be formulated for each brain-injured person before discharge from the hospital. The approach of rehabilitation should be comprehensive and intensive. Follow-up of the patients is essential if rehabilitative gains are to be sustained.

Though there are common traits, each brain injury manifests itself differently, so any intervention strategy will need to be tailored to address these differences. Uniformity or a package-based module is not a desired regimen for intervention as patients have been found to benefit if the tasks are tailor-made. Therefore, while tailoring the tasks, the therapist should keep in mind environmental factors, preinjury history, site of the injury, and severity of the injury. There should be tangible and interactive routines, collaborative decision making with other professionals and family members should be made part of the ongoing program. There is no single "right" or "wrong" solution. The therapist should also be ready with several tasks and plans—sometimes the best one can do is to keep trying various plans since what works today won't work tomorrow.

A holistic approach to neurorehabilitation would involve exploring and handling every aspect of individual functioning that has become impaired and reintegrating the individual back into society at the highest level possible. A plethora of strategies have been developed to enhance individual functioning in physical, cognitive, and behavioral realms of functioning. Often, a multidisciplinary approach comprising neurologists, physiatrists, neuropsychologists, and speech and occupational therapists is involved in various aspects of rehabilitation. Neuropsychologists are intimately involved in helping the patient and family deal with the trauma, assessing and enhancing the cognitive functions, and providing a blueprint for individual's gainful employment and

Neuropsychological Rehabilitation-Principles and Applications.
DOI: http://dx.doi.org/10.1016/B978-0-12-416046-0.00003-1

engagement in society. Whether compensatory or remedial, a variety of techniques are utilized, ranging from cognitive retraining to behavior therapy approaches such as operant conditioning, contingency management, shaping, and cognitive restructuring.

There is now empirical evidence across the world that comprehensive neuropsychological rehabilitation yields the best outcomes. Goldstein [1] found intensive rehabilitation effective in helping many people return to a meaningful life after a serious brain injury. It is a practical approach using the strengths of the patient to develop coping abilities. It is also an educational process, which helps develop adaptive strategies for coping. Training with the use of compensatory aids and systems helps reduce the handicap and encourages independence. Better communication and understanding between professionals and family members can make the family feel "part of the team" and allow professionals and family members to benefit from each other's knowledge of the individual with brain injury.

To attain optimal rehabilitation benefit of the brain-injured person, it is essential to coordinate and integrate the cognitive remedial training (i.e., those interventions that are aimed at making it possible for the person to compensate for specific intellectual and behavioral impairments) along with the other clinical interventions (e.g., helping the person accept the disability, restoring a sense of hope; motivating and improving morale, teaching the person ways of adjusting to misfortune and new roles, exercising appropriate social judgment, and having a positive outlook on life).

It has been found that even when the physical factors resolve, cognitive, emotional, and behavioral problems persist; these are the greatest source of stress to caregivers and obstruct the patient's return to work [2]. A study has indicated that about 40% of those hospitalized with a traumatic brain injury (TBI) had at least one unmet need for services one year after the injury [1a] noted that about 40% of those hospitalized with a traumatic brain injury (TBI) had at least one unmet need for services one year after the injury. The most frequent unmet needs were improving memory and problem solving, managing stress and emotional outbursts, controlling one's temper, and improving job skills. It is thus clear that the role of the clinician does not end with treating the medical and cognitive consequences of a TBI. Emotional, personality, and behavioral changes after TBI can lead to serious and long-lasting impairments in social [3] and occupational functioning, often preventing return to earlier work status [2]. The emotional/behavioral problems significantly affect recovery, rehabilitation outcome, and reintegration into the community [4]. The consequences of TBI also have important implications for quality of life and subjective satisfaction of the individual. In an extensive report on TBI in India, Gururaj et al. [5] observed that quality of life was poor in 30% of the injured 2 years postdischarge. Another study showed that employment, social integration, and mood status were associated with better life satisfaction in the second year after a TBI [6]. It has been suggested that early detection and management of emotional distress is paramount in enhancing long-term outcomes following TBI [4].

In the earliest stages of recovery, survivors and family members are often bewildered by the patient's behavior. Prior to the injury, the patient was a responsible adult and now they find a problematic child among them. The physical disability is better accepted by significant others than the behavioral and the cognitive disability. Hence, clinicians can use counseling to effectively educate caregivers and patients about orientation, attention, memory, sleep, behavioral, emotional, and self-confidence problems and to prepare the patient and the family members for the rehabilitation process.

For cognitive retraining to be effective, the following three factors should be considered:

1. Cognitive tasks and mediation
2. Psychological services
3. Other services.

## Cognitive Tasks and Mediation

The overall aim of rehabilitation should be to help patients adapt and come to terms with their new self and to achieve peace of mind in their new life situation through realistic goals and aspirations. They should be helped to operate in the real-world at the maximum level of which they are capable, and they should be provided with whatever ongoing support is necessary to maintain that level of operation. This sort of rehabilitation needs to be carried out on an individualized basis and follow a comprehensive approach, taking into account all aspects of the person's life.

As most of the people afflicted with TBI are in the age range of 20s to 40s, with a normal life expectancy, it is important that they get help in returning to some sort of realistic, productive activity which they find satisfying. This means, among other things, informing and educating concerned staff at the educational institution, employment service, and employers about the nature of brain injury and its effects so that patients get appropriate help and support.

### Cognitive Tasks

The first step in the rehabilitation process is to carry out a detailed interview with the patient and significant others. The second step involves administering a comprehensive neuropsychological assessment to arrive at a specific neuropsychological profile of the individual. The third step is based on identifying the strengths and weakness such that cognitive tasks for retraining can be developed. The tasks should be simple, practical, empirically grounded in theory, and they should allow for measurement in terms of time and error. Tasks should allow for modification in terms of complexity as the retaining proceeds. It should be tailor-made for individual patients. The cognitive tasks are given to the patient everyday for an hour. The tasks are administered in graded difficulty, and saturation cueing method is followed. The cognitive tasks administered should reach an optimum level, and once the level is maintained for 3–4 days, the task difficulty is increased. Constant changes are made depending on the patient's performance, and psychological mediation of behavior is done using principles of reinforcement and contingency management.

Patients initially ask numerous questions, and answering these questions is very important, since this can facilitate patients' involvement in the cognitive rehabilitation process. This is the first step toward improvement (Figure 3.1).

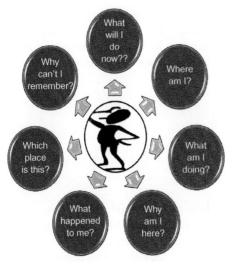

**Figure 3.1** First step toward improvement.

## Mediation

Feuerstein's Instrumental Enrichment Program [7] is a cognitive intervention program in which a mediated learning process is used as a part of the cognitive rehabilitation.

### Mediation of Meaning

The tasks given to the patient may be very simple in the initial stages. The patient may not understand the reasons for the tasks being administered. Hence answering the questions Why? What? What for? Why not? Why for? and so on is crucial for the sustenance of the rehabilitation process. If possible, the tasks should be explained on a theoretical basis along with the brain domains they address. A detailed behavioral analysis of the patient including behavioral excesses and deficits should be made. If a behavior is desirable, the patient should be positively reinforced; if it is an undesirable behavior, negative reinforcement techniques should be used. The significance of each activity that is carried out should be explained to both the patient and significant others as this can foster improvement in the patient and enhance confidence in the treatment. In the initial stages of the rehabilitation, basic cognitive deficits in attention, comprehension, judgment, orientation, and motivation can cause communication difficulties. Hence, the use of paralinguistic modes (e.g., body language and changes in amplitude, tone, and tempo of the voice) and, depending on the need, alteration of bodily movements can be emphasized by the therapist.

### Mediation of Motivation

Motivation is a very important factor in cognitive rehabilitation. Most of the patients with brain injury are amotivated in the initial stages. To improve motivation, the patient should be encouraged to understand the tasks given, and reinforcements should be provided to enhance performance. The therapist should ensure that the patient has comprehended the task well and the improvements are getting generalized to situations of daily living. Once this is done, the patient should be encouraged to experience success on the tasks given and it should be explained how this has an implication on activities of daily living. If the patient fails to understand, the explanation should be repeated at several sessions in the cognitive rehabilitation process, and at every instance the patient should be offered enough assistance for success. However, the inputs from the therapist should be limited in order to facilitate more action on the patient's part, thus promoting independence.

## Mediation of Regulation of Control of Behavior

It is well known that behavioral problems are evident in patients with brain injury. Some kinds of emotional, personality, and behavioral changes have been reported in 85% of injured persons and 87% of relatives of the injured [2]. The most common changes in emotional/behavioral functioning following a TBI include depressed mood, fluctuations in mood state, frustration and anger outbursts, reduced tolerance to stress, difficulties in emotional expression and regulation, poor motivation and initiation [4], altered sense of humor including inappropriate or facetious comments, impulsivity, rigidity and stubbornness, reduced or inappropriate sexual behavior, excessive eating, spending, and talking, and psychotic symptoms [8]. In addition, psychiatric disorders can be a result of TBI. A review [9] summarized that anxiety has been reported in up to 70% of individuals with TBI, while the prevalence rates of anxiety disorder following a TBI have been reported to be between 20% and 30%. Depression and psychotic disorders are also a frequent consequence of TBI.

Most often patients do not have insight into these problems, which can result in interpersonal problems in social and occupational spheres. Family members should understand that these behavioral problems are a result of the brain injury. Cognitive tasks and behavioral techniques should be used simultaneously in order to obtain gains in various domains of living. The patient should be taught to practice from response inappropriateness to response appropriateness and to reflect and work on his/her abilities. The therapist should emphasize the importance of internal locus of control.

## Mediation of Sharing Behavior

Due to brain injury, patients' social activities are affected; they are confined to home setting, and relatives may find it embarrassing to accompany patients to social events. Educating the patient's relatives regarding the need for social and interpersonal opportunities is important. Explaining the importance of sharing the process and experience is crucial. In this way, the patient's self-esteem may be restored.

## Mediation of Individual and Psychological Differentiations

Brain-injured patients not only suffer from poor self-esteem but also lack self-confidence. Help should be provided so that the patient can become an articulated, differentiated self. Patients become dependent on others physically, emotionally, and financially. Trust and acceptance should be emphasized in order to restore confidence in patients. Therapists should also help patients make future plans in terms of planning and goal seeking and setting, and steps in achieving the plan should be emphasized.

# Psychological Services

## Psychosocial Factors

Studies indicate that patients with TBI face numerous psychosocial problems [10,11]. The impact of the consequences of the brain injury on both the individual's system of social activities and relationships, and upon others within their social system is found to be alarming. Reduction in the size of the social system, changes in the nature of relationships, changes in roles, and increased financial burdens are highlighted as imposing significant burdens on both the individual and the family.

Many studies have reported long-term psychosocial difficulties in TBI, including social isolation, especially among those who are unemployed and have few leisure activities [12]; lack of social contact outside the immediate family [13–15]; inability to engage in appropriate social interaction [16–18]; inability to find a companion or spouse; and dependency within the family [19].

Caregivers often use emotion-focused techniques in dealing with the illness, which in turn has a negative effect on the patient's improvement. Hence, there is a need to consider the subjective understanding and experience of the brain-injury survivor and the family or caregiver. Thus, a greater emphasis is needed on a biopsychosocial approach to understand the consequences of brain injury and in particular the emotional consequences. The therapist should consider physical and cognitive impairments, functional difficulties, and social and cultural factors in making treatment plans in order to enhance patient's engagement and involvement in therapy, it is important that the therapist keeps him aware and informed at every stage of therapy. Functional rehabilitative efforts are likely to have a positive impact on emotional well-being through improved quality of life. Modified cognitive behavioral therapy may provide both a system and a set of interventions that are particularly appropriate for brain-injured patients.

## Psychotherapy

Brain injury has both neurological and psychiatric consequences [20]. Neuropsychological rehabilitation is concerned not only with restoring cognitive functions, but also with personality, emotion, and awareness. Since the brain is the mediator of these functions [21], psychotherapy in the rehabilitation setting is often indicated. It should target the issues of self-awareness, egocentricity, empathy, coping, and adjustment. The individual is frequently reminded of the losses he/she has faced when he/she hears about the changes in others' lives [22] such as getting a job, a promotion, marriage, and birth of children. The judgments and reactions of others and their effect on the individual's sense of self are also important factors. Individuals with TBI often feel that family and friends are either cold and unsympathetic or condescending toward their abilities and adjustment. Other factors associated with distress are loss of old friendships and an inability to make new ones, changes in living arrangements, and leisure activities being reduced by half after the injury [2]. As one client with severe agnosia for objects and faces, achromatopsia, topographical disorientation, and alexia said, "I used to love shopping for vegetables, but now, they all look like strange lumps to me, and I can't tell which is which. I could go to a dance or theatre performance, I enjoy that, but I can't see the color of the costumes, or understand the expressions on the faces of the performers. My favorite pastimes were reading and driving, and I can't do either of that now."

In addition, TBI has a profound impact on sense of identity—the individual is no longer the same as he/she was preinjury and finds that he/she has to adjust to changed abilities, roles, and expectations [23]. Due to these problems, depression is very common in individuals after TBI. Further, one study showed that individuals who had difficulty in achieving reintegration and resumption of preinjury roles were more likely to endorse external locus of control indices such as "powerful others" and "chance" [24], leading to a vicious circle of disengagement from rehabilitation goals.

Anxiety syndromes, specifically acute stress disorder, posttraumatic stress disorder (PTSD), panic disorder, generalized anxiety disorder, and obsessive–compulsive disorder, have also been reported after TBI. Anxiety symptoms may be attributed to trauma to the amygdala that, like the hippocampus, is prone to injury because of its mesial temporal location. Limited data exists regarding the effectiveness of psychopharmacologic agents for the treatment of anxiety disorders in patients with TBI. Bryant et al. [25] suggested that early treatment of acute stress disorder with cognitive behavioral therapy might prevent the development of PTSD.

The famous case of Phineas Gage illustrates the personality changes commonly observed after TBI, specifically frontal lobe injury. One study found that a personality disorder developed in 23.3% of patients as a result of TBI [26]. Aggression and impulsivity are commonly encountered after brain trauma, especially in the acute/subacute period. Orbitofrontal injury is strongly correlated with impulsive aggression. Several treatment strategies have been proposed in patients with TBI. Atypical antipsychotics, Selective Serotonin Reuptake Inhibitors (SSRI), lamotrigine, and buspirone along with psychotherapy also have been used for managing posttraumatic aggression [27,28]. Although the development of chronic psychotic symptoms, such as hallucinations and delusions, is a relatively infrequent result of TBI, these symptoms are not uncommonly observed in the acute phase after TBI. When present, these symptoms can be quite debilitating. These posttraumatic psychotic symptoms are thought to be caused by prefrontal and/or temporal lobe injury [29,30].

In order for psychotherapy to circumvent the cognitive problems that are common after TBI, the use of concrete images and concepts, employing drawing, music, and popular literature has been recommended [31]. Cognitive therapies focusing on identity, acceptance, and facilitation of "normal" adjustment using techniques such as anger management, problem solving, assertiveness, and social and communication skills training are observed to be particularly helpful. Social skills training may be focused toward social nuances such as initiating conversations, choosing appropriate topics for conversation, understanding personal boundaries (such as not revealing personal information to strangers, not standing too close to another person), taking turns speaking, making eye contact, modulating pitch and tone, and interpreting nonverbal cues (such as when another person wants to end the conversation). Anger management may include withdrawing from a potentially anger-provoking situation, distraction strategies, relaxation, using assertive rather than aggressive communication, understanding the consequences of giving in to anger, etc. Use of behavior modification strategies such as star charts, token economy, and time out is particularly helpful in increasing desirable behaviors and decreasing undesirable or maladaptive ones in individuals with TBI. There is some evidence for the role of cognitive behavior therapy in reducing anxiety and depression [32]. Moderate support exists for behavioral interventions in children and adults, prompting recommendation of such interventions as a practice guideline [33].

## Financial and Employment Issues

Vocational rehabilitation poses a daunting challenge for professionals engaged in successful reintegration of the patient into society. It is estimated that nearly 1 million persons are injured, 200,000 people die and nearly 1 million require rehabilitation services every year in India [5]. A majority of these individuals are children, adolescents, and young adults ranging from 15 to 25 years [34,35]. These figures are indicative of the huge disease care burden that TBI exerts on the society. Brain-injured survivors are no longer able to compete in the job market at the level at which they were premorbidly functioning. Brain injury causes cognitive impairments and, as a result, it has a bearing on occupational functioning, including poor time management, organizational difficulties, and social inappropriateness. Since the victims are often young men, the economic status of the entire family is affected. On the one hand, there is the increased burden of the health-care costs (medicines, physiotherapy, and other rehabilitation service charges); on the other hand, there is a reduction in the family income when the earning member becomes disabled after TBI. In such a scenario, the primary goal of the rehabilitation professional is to enable the patient to become both physically and financially independent.

In financial rehabilitation, it is important to consider factors that influence the degree to which an individual can be functionally reintegrated into the society. These include injury-related factors such as the degree of severity and disability caused by the injury that prevents the individual from attaining functional independence; age at time of injury—the older the individual at time of injury, the less likely return to work [36–38]; preinjury education level and marital status—if not a high-school graduate and if single, the less likely return to work [37,39]; cognitive factors such as attention deficits, memory impairments that interfere with day-to-day functioning of the individual; personality-related factors such as passivity, pessimism, low

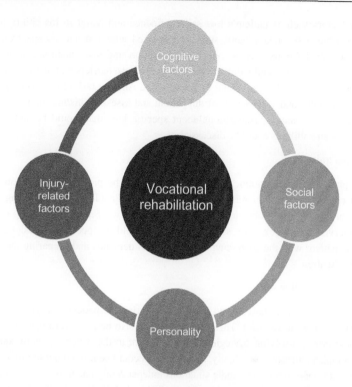

**Figure 3.2** Multiple components of vocational rehabilitation.

self-confidence, and poor body image; and social factors such as family support, financial status of the family, and ability to maintain social interactions.

These factors can be shown in the form of a diagram (Figure 3.2). All these factors mutually interact with each other and consequently influence the vocational rehabilitation of an individual. For example, the severity of an injury would have specific repercussions on the cognitive functioning of the individual, which would further impact the psychological state of the individual (causing personality changes or making the individual feel anxious and depressed because of his disability), and it would ultimately impact the overall family functioning, thereby leading to burnout of the caretakers. The process of vocational rehabilitation can be divided into three major phases:

**1.** Prevocational counseling

This is the first and the most significant phase of rehabilitation. It is important to pay special consideration to the timing of this phase, as too premature or too delayed a beginning could pose challenges in reintegration of the individual into the workforce. Ideally, only after the patient has achieved basic improvement in physical, cognitive, and behavioral aspects of the illness should vocational plans be put forth. At this stage, there could be situational barriers such as a paucity of suitable jobs or difficulty in returning to the earlier workplace, personality factors such as patient's low self-confidence and belief in his ability to resume work or to achieve secondary gains such as increased attention and escape from responsibilities, and social factors such as poor family support and inadequate social interactions. Prevocational counseling should aim at overcoming all these barriers and instilling motivation and a sense of hope in individual about rejoining work. Another task of this phase is identifying specific strengths and weaknesses of the patient and assessing his/her interests and skills. Based on these assessments, suggestions about specific jobs that would be suitable for the patient's needs and abilities could be discussed.

**2.** Vocational training

In this phase of rehabilitation, an individual needs to be prepared for the job situation. Vocational counselors or other rehabilitation professionals could assist in looking for suitable jobs, applying for these jobs, and preparing for interviews. Simulated training in the form of mock interviews or mock work settings and tasks could be specifically designed so as to acquaint the patient with the work environment and its demands and preparing them to enter the real-life situation.

**3.** Monitoring and follow-up

The third and the final phase would involve monitoring the patient's progress at the workplace through follow-up sessions. These sessions could also be utilized to provide brief interventions, and problem-solving strategies could be taught to the patient so as to equip him to deal with complex situations. Gradually, these sessions could be phased out in order to provide individuals with opportunities to handle situations independently and thus become self-reliant.

The above plan could be integrated into the holistic rehabilitation plan for a particular individual and could be executed by professionals involved in providing care to the patient.

## Family Therapy

A majority of the people affected by TBI are young people, with normal life expectancy. They tend to drift aimlessly through life. The quality of their life is very low. Having a person with a head injury in the family places a great burden and stress on close family members, whose lives are changed forever. Clare et al. [40] assert that family members feel that they suddenly have a different person among them, who looks the same but behaves quite differently and is unaware of what has happened to him/her. It is in some respects like having lost an adult son or daughter, or a partner, and gained an argumentative child in the family. But they are not children. The family will need support and education on how the head injury has affected the patient, and how best to cope with the situation. They will need guidance on sources of informed help and advice. They may also need counseling because their stress levels tend to increase with time.

It has to be recognized by the family members that, although the most obvious and rapid improvements take place in about the first 2 years, significant improvement can occur over many years. However, there will generally be residual deficits that will remain with the person for the rest of their life and with which they will need ongoing help.

Medical and rehabilitation professionals often become so enmeshed in the overt physical, cognitive, and behavioral impairments that some of the implicit yet basic aspects of individual functioning are ignored. One such aspect is sexual functioning of the individual who has recovered from the physical and cognitive limitations of the injury/disease but is unable to lead a normal, healthy life.

## Marital and Sexual Issues

Sexuality is considered to be an intricate yet vital aspect of human existence. It goes beyond the physical union of two individuals and includes the cognitive, affective, and interpersonal components of behavior. It is considered to be an interface of mind and body. Most rehabilitation programs consider independent daily living and some degree of occupational engagement as the end target. However, as the individual begins to improve in his physical, cognitive, and emotional aspects, his understanding of his overall functioning as well as significant others' expectations of them begin to increase. In such a scenario, either the individual himself or the spouse will often become perplexed about matters related to sexual functioning. Since rehabilitation is a slow process and extends often to months after the injury/disease, individuals begin to have a low self-image, perceive themselves as weak and dependent, and are uncertain of their capabilities.

According to one study, almost half of all intimate relationships and one-third of marriages break down following a TBI [2]. TBI has an impact on the sexual/marital domain in three ways: it alters the individual's sexual functioning and emotional responsiveness; the sexual/emotional changes in the injured individual affect the partner; the partner's reactions to these changes in turn affect the injured and the relationship as a whole (Figure 3.3).

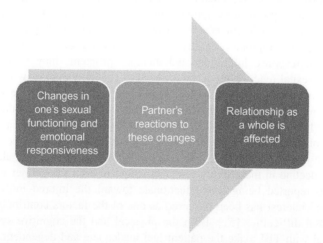

**Figure 3.3 Process of change in sexual functioning after injury or illness.**

Sexuality was reported as one of the least satisfying domains 10 years after TBI [2]. Reviewing sexual functioning after TBI, Zasler and Martelli [41] summarized that across studies, approximately half of individuals with TBI experience some form of altered sexual functioning, such as reduced libido, erectile dysfunction, alteration in sexual preferences, or preoccupation with sex. Degree of physical independence has been observed as one of the predictors of sexual adjustment [42]. One study reported that frequency of sexual intercourse decreased for 75% of female patients and for 55% of male patients [43].

TBIs are significantly associated with sexual disturbances. Blackerby [44] emphasized that since most head injuries occur in the age group of 20–30, there is a disruption in sexual relationships. In adolescents, it leads to an arrest of the sexual self-concept. Most often, damage to brain structures such as the frontal lobes, hypo-thalamus, amygdale, and septic nuclei can lead to impairments in sexual functioning [45,46]. Sexual problems frequently reported in men posttraumatic injury are 41% report low sexual desire [47], 30% report erectile dysfunction, and 40% report ejaculation problems [42]. Women with TBI report reduced sexual desire (35%), lubrication problems (26%), reduced or no experience of orgasm (40%), and 50% of women report decreased to nil frequency of sexual activity postinjury [42,48].

TBI has an impact on the sexual functioning of an individual both directly and indirectly. The direct or the primary causes of sexual problems after TBI include lesions or abnormalities in frontal or limbic structures that are considered to be the seat of sexual urges, motivation, and performance. The indirect or the secondary causes of sexual dysfunction post-TBI include feelings of inadequacy, depression, anxiety, chronic pain, or the effects of medications. Often the physical symptoms such as weakness in hands or legs, chronic pain, tremors, or sensitivity to touch may cause clumsiness in lovemaking and increased pain or other unpleasant experi-ences during sexual intercourse. Fatigue also could complicate matters, as this would decrease involvement, reduce satisfaction, and lower the desire to engage in sexual activity. Since these physical symptoms are more prominent in the initial phase of injury, the patient and the partners refrain from engaging in sexual interactions. Along with these physical symptoms, cognitive symptoms such as decreased attention span, impairments in response inhibition, and memory problems may have a negative impact on the sexual functioning of the individual. The individual may feel distracted during the sexual act, may show an increased rush to reach intercourse without any foreplay, and might repetitively ask for sexual interaction due to forgetfulness.

The injured individual's sexual functioning has a significant effect on the partner. Almost half of the spouses interviewed in one study reported having no sexual out-let due to the partner's problems with sexual functioning [49]. Wives also reported a significant decline in their ability to achieve orgasm after the partner was injured. Partners also reported being less affectionate toward the injured individual [50]. Altered sexual interest has been observed as one of the factors contributing to fam-ily and marital difficulties [51]. Both the physical and the cognitive symptoms of the individual with TBI make the patient feel inadequate and dependent. Often, the spouse (in most cases women) assumes the role of a parent and provides nurturance and care to the patient. Gosling and Oddy [52] investigated the quality of the marital and sexual relationships in 18 heterosexual couples. These couples were assessed 1–7 years after the male partner had suffered a severe head injury. The methodology of the study included both quantitative and qualitative methods. The results indicated that there was a significant change in sexual satisfaction following the injury. Women reported low sexual satisfaction as compared to their male counterparts. It was found that women experienced significant role changes, often a role reversal, with many comparing their new role to that of a parent with responsibilities for managing the house and the family and making vital decisions. They also reported this role to be incompatible with that of a sexual partner.

Speech, cognitive, and social deficits following TBI may contribute to poorer communication in the injured individual that may impact the quality of marital interactions; however, there is also some suggestion that communication problems may affect larger social contexts without disturbing the marital sphere [53]. Blais and Boisvert also found that an effective attitude to problems, infrequent use of avoidance coping strategies, and positive perception of spouse's communication skills were most significantly associated with psychological adjustment and marital satisfaction following a TBI. Further, the personal characteristics of the spouse contributed to the marital satisfaction of the injured partner. Another study demonstrated that age, gender, ethnicity, severity, and time since injury were factors predicting marital stability [54]. Other issues relating to the partner, such as caregiver's burden, anger, and guilt about taking time off may also affect the relationship [2].

As the physical and cognitive symptoms tend to improve and the patient improves his functioning, awareness, and insight about his condition also increases. In most cases, there is a gnawing sense of doubt about complete recovery and uncertainty regarding one's future. The individual attempts to adjust to the role changes that have ensued in the family as a consequence of his debility. There is reduced self-esteem, loss of confidence in one's ability, and poor body image, resulting in feelings of anxiety and depression. These states lower the sexual drive and reduce the motivation to engage in sexual activity, and the individual feels withdrawn and aloof. In such situations, if the communication patterns between the spouses are not healthy, this could lead to significant relationship difficulties, with the patient feeling depressed and inadequate and the spouse feeling rejected and burned out in the role of caretaker and frustrated due to lack of sexual interaction. Thus, the interaction of these physical, cognitive, and psychological factors can adversely impact sexual functioning.

Having discussed the impact and gravity of TBI on sexual function, it becomes imperative to provide a management plan for addressing this issue in holistic rehabilitation. The first and the most significant step involves sensitizing rehabilitation professionals to inquire about any sexual problems in their routine investigations of the patients. Most often, in our country, there exists a social barrier that prevents discussion of such intimate matters. Not just the patient and his spouse but the treating professional may feel somewhat hesitant to explore for any sexual difficulties following the injury/disease. Thus, the first step in rehabilitation of sexual functioning would involve opening up the communication channels—for the treating professional as well as the spouse.

The PLISSIT model given by Annon [55] could be used as a guiding framework in this regard. The first step involves providing *permission* to clients to discuss their sexual issues and concerns. When the patients are able to discuss their issues with a professional, much of their anxiety and uncertainty about their capabilities gets resolved and they feel relaxed. The second step involves providing *limited information* to the patient and spouse wherein their specific difficulties, concerns, and myths are addressed and the professional provides corrective guidance on such issues. The third step involves providing *specific suggestions* to address the particular problems and concerns of each couple. Patients with brain injury often have concerns regarding their ability to perform, and they may feel inadequate because of physical weakness and fatigue. The suggestions may include specific physical exercises for dealing with weakness, specific attention-enhancement strategies for dealing with cognitive symptoms affecting sexual functioning, and specific inputs to enhance self-esteem and body image. The final step in this framework involves providing *intensive therapy* to those individuals in whom sexual difficulties are complicated by comorbid anxiety or depression or where the overall relationship is characterized by conflicts and disruption. A comprehensive history of the couple is taken, and the factors escalating the spiral of conflicts are recognized and effectively handled in therapy.

Behavioral therapy techniques such as imagery, body exploration, and sensitization training for arousal and orgasmic dysfunction in men and women, and the squeeze technique for premature ejaculation are recommended. Behavior modification techniques may be important for reducing hypersexuality. For individuals without an active sexual partner, masturbation with appropriate regard for privacy is proposed as an option. The need for counseling for the individual and the family about problems in sexual functioning has been emphasized, with a frank and open discussion of options, do's and don'ts, and sensitivity to moral and religious beliefs [41].

## Other Professional Services

Neuropsychological rehabilitation should be carried out by involving an interdisciplinary team of specialists including speech therapists, occupational therapists, staff nurses, physiotherapists, physiatrists, psychiatrists, ophthalmologists, ENT specialists, general physicians, etc., whenever the need is felt. Rehabilitation needs to be looked at from a multidisciplinary perspective and should target the physical, cognitive, interpersonal, and social impairments. It thus requires a team of professionals who can provide their expert services in each area and help the individual to regain his optimal functioning. It is imperative that these professionals share their inputs in order to enhance each other's role and functions (Figure 3.4).

The authors would like to conclude this chapter by providing two case vignettes that illustrate the concepts discussed in the chapter.

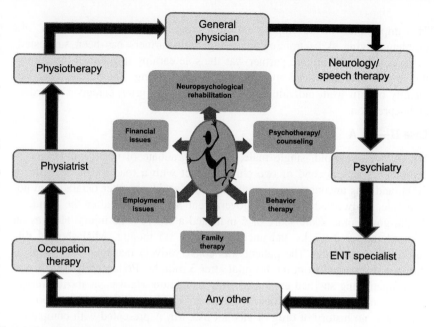

**Figure 3.4** A holistic approach to rehabilitation.

### Case I—Mr. Mukund (name changed)

Mr. Mukund was a 35-year-old advertising executive who sustained a TBI in an automobile accident while on a work-related trip. He was left with severe deficits in attention and new learning, along with slurred speech and hemiparesis. His wife, who had always been a homemaker, was forced to take up a teaching job, besides caring for their two children. Mukund also developed a preoccupation with bowel and bladder functions, making his wife wait for hours while he insisted on relieving himself, even though he had just been taken to the toilet. Whenever he made sexual advances, his wife avoided him. "I simply can't do it with him anymore. I have spent so much time taking him back and forth to the toilet, and helping him clean up, that it's difficult to feel sexually attracted to him. But do you think it will help him? If it will, I can force myself to go through with it." Before the injury, Mukund had been the dominant partner in the relationship, and his current "weak" role disturbed the wife. Before rehabilitation began, she had often prodded him to use his left hand, to try harder to walk, urging him to "be a man!" She was convinced that if he could only start walking again, he would get back his confidence and resume work.

Mukund's case illustrates the need to address multiple aspects of the sexual and marital domain. Educating the family about the nature and consequences of a TBI is crucial in modifying their expectations of the recovery process.

The importance of developing tailored programs for communication and problem-solving skills training involving both partners has been suggested. In cases where the injured partner was the sole earning member of the family, the spouse may also need vocational guidance/training. The partner may frequently benefit from individual therapy to deal with grief, caregiver's burden, and depression.

### Case II—Mr. A

Mr. A, a 24-year-old, single male, B.Com. graduate of upper-middle socio-economic status, second of two children, met with a road traffic accident in 2008, and was unconscious immediately after accident; other details were not available. He was admitted in a government hospital 10h after the accident. A Glasgow Coma Scale score of 6 indicated a severe head injury. He was on a ventilator for 2 weeks and unconscious for 1½ months. MRI showed diffused cerebral edema. The patient was conservatively managed with medication and discharged from the hospital after 3 months. Premorbidly, Mr. A was high functioning and had graduated with distinction. He was an above-average student from childhood. No history of mental or physical illness was reported. There was no history of drug or alcohol use. Mr. A presented with complaints of motor slowness, inability to attend to information, would easily get tired, memory disturbances (would forget incidents within a day, would forget names and faces of familiar people), had difficulty naming things, had word-finding difficulty and fluctuations in his mood with irritability; anger outbursts were also reported.

Mr. A was referred to the neuropsychology unit for neuropsychological assessment and rehabilitation.

## Neuropsychological Assessment and Rehabilitation

A written informed consent was obtained from the patient and neuropsychological assessment and retraining were carried out.

Neuropsychological assessment was carried out to generate a profile to understand his strengths and deficits. Cognitive functioning of the patient was compared with normative data derived from a group of 540 normal healthy volunteers [56]. Based on the number of test variables falling below the 15th percentile, the severity of cognitive impairment was established.

Precognitive retraining neuropsychological assessment showed deficits in attention, fluency, working memory, planning, verbal and visual learning, and memory. His neuropsychological profile was indicative of dorsolateral prefrontal cortex and bilateral temporal lobe involvement.

The neuropsychological rehabilitation was tailor-made to improve or restore his attention, memory, organizing, reasoning and understanding, problem solving,

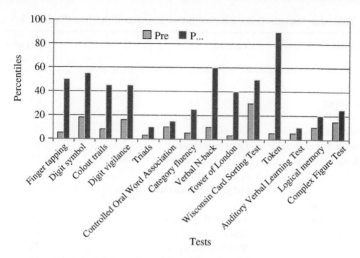

**Figure 3.5** Comparison of test scores pre- and postintervention.

and decision making. Initially, basic cognitive functions were addressed. Cognitive retraining was carried out for a period of 4 months over 65 sessions, everyday for 1 h. Principles of saturation cueing were followed. The tasks were given in increasing difficulty levels and were designed with provision for scoring error and time. Patient's issues were addressed at every sphere; a biological, psychological, and social approach was adopted.

Following the precognitive retraining, neuropsychological assessment deficits were found in the domains of attention, verbal memory, visual memory, facial recognition, reasoning ability, planning, sequencing, word-finding difficulty, and irritability.

Results indicated significant improvement in these functions postintervention (Figure 3.5). Cognitive retraining commenced with the target of improving the basic functions; attention tasks were given to improve both focused and sustained attention, and response inhibition tasks were started from the first session onward. Patient started showing improvement on these tasks, and hence, tasks for working memory and word-finding difficulty were introduced from the 22nd session. In the 30th session, verbal memory tasks were introduced. Patient showed significant improvement on all these tasks and in his day-to-day functioning, which was reported by the significant others. At the 40th session, tasks were designed to improve patient's ability for facial recognition and emotional regulation as these continued to remain areas of concern. Overall, patient underwent cognitive retraining for 65 sessions over a period of 4 months. Improvements were seen on the tasks as well as in his everyday functioning. Symptom rating was done with patient and mother after every 10 sessions on a visual analog scale of 1–10 (1 indicates no impairment; 10 indicates severe impairment).

Postcognitive retraining assessment showed improvement in all the domains except in set shifting (Table 3.1).

**Table 3.1** Various Tasks and Number of Sessions to Address Each Deficit

| Functions | Tasks | Number of Sessions |
|---|---|---|
| Attention | | |
|   Sustained | Grain sorting | 65 |
|   Focused | Number cancellation | 40 |
|   Directed | Coloring | 40 |
| Word-finding difficulty | Common words | 20 |
| Working memory | Digits backward and forward | 25 |
| Verbal | Jumbled sentences | 30 |
| Visual | Reversing clocks and figures | 30 |
| Verbal memory | Temporal encoding | 49 |
| Visual memory | Spatial encoding | 40 |
| | Visual sketch pad | 34 |
| | Visual memory for meaningful designs | 45 |
| Emotional regulation | Statue test | 15 |
| | Responding to cues | 10 |
| | Depicting emotions on instructions | 16 |
| | Story | 15 |
| Face recognition | Faces with distinct marks | 35 |
| | Faces without distinct marks | 29 |

## Process Issues During Cognitive Retraining

Cognitive retraining began with an explanation of the tasks and their rationale. The patient did not understand the implicit reasons for the tasks and hence resisted by repeatedly asking Why? Why not? What for?

Hence, the relevance of the tasks to certain behaviors of the patient was focused and explained. The significance of each activity was elaborated in detail. Initially, the therapist used paralinguistic modes (e.g., body language, changes in amplitude of the voice, and alteration of movements). The importance of motivation in the tasks was explained and the patient was helped in orientation toward the search for meaning. It was ensured that the meaning had been registered and connections related to other events were highlighted. It helped him to experience the success and to see its impact toward generalization on day-to-day functioning.

Since the patient had low self-esteem, a feeling of competence was emphasized, and this was accomplished through helping the patient experience success or perceiving the positive value of previously experienced encounters. The patient also exhibited poor inhibitory control, and hence, this was achieved through regulation of control of behavior from inhibition to internal control, nonreflective to self-reflection, response inappropriateness to response appropriateness. Due to poor inhibitory control, patient was confined at home, since the significant other felt embarrassed in social situations; hence, the need to go outside by himself with the objective

**Table 3.2** Comparison of Visual Analog Scale Scores Pre- and Postintervention

| Symptoms | Preneuropsychological Rehabilitation | Postneuropsychological Rehabilitation |
|---|---|---|
| Motor slowness | 10 | 0 |
| Inability to attend, would easily get tired | 8 | 0 |
| Memory disturbances: forget incidents within a day, would forget names and faces of familiar people | 9 | 2 |
| Unable to name things, word-finding difficulty | 10 | 2 |
| Fluctuations in mood: irritability, anger outburst | 9 | 1 |

of participating with others and making others participate with the patient was explained. The meaning of sharing the process and experience was explained and amplified.

Patient was helped to become independent in his activities and thinking; trust and acceptance was emphasized with the significant others. Emotional affective relationship was enhanced by belonging and feeling of acceptance by others. Mediated goal seeking, setting, planning, and achieving behavior were also assisted.

## Counseling and Therapy

Individual therapy as and when required with the patient was carried out for 31 sessions. Issues regarding the adjustment with his mother and his personal requirements, which were at times unreasonable, were dealt with. Supportive therapy was carried out with the parents for nine sessions. Mother was the decision maker in the family and after patient's injury she began to treat him like a child. As the patient improved, he resented mother's authority and control, which led to significant distress in their relationship. Since the patient was very demanding, the parents found it difficult to handle him; they were educated about the problems and were taught to handle him appropriately. Individual and joint sessions (11 sessions) were carried out with predominant emphasis on their interpersonal functioning. Other family issues such as how to handle the patient during his anger outbursts and adjustments with other family members such as patient's sister were also addressed during the sessions. Environmental restructuring was also suggested as the patient did not want to face his friends and relatives.

Rating was obtained on a 10-point visual analog scale by the patient and mother (Table 3.2).

Cognitive retraining is useful in head injury. Cognitive retraining along with other adjunct therapy seeks to retrain and reeducate patients to compromise and cope with existing problems. It integrates the patient back into society at the highest level of functioning possible.

## Conclusions

- Cognitive tasks and mediation, psychological services, and services by other professionals are important ingredients in holistic rehabilitation.
- Brain injury-related changes often have negative impact on relationships. Major issues arise from cognitive, emotional, and behavioral problems.
- Individuals who sustain a brain injury must cope with increased dependence on family and friends, as well as social rejection caused by societal stereotypes of disability.
- Vocational rehabilitation should be an important goal, and professionals should plan and provide the required support.
- Holistic rehabilitation requires careful planning and immense skill and flexibility on the part of the professionals to tailor it to individual needs.

## References

[1] Goldstein, K. (1995). *The organism: A holistic approach to biology from pathological data in man.* New York: Zone Books.

[1a] Corrigan, J. D., Whiteneck, G., & Mellick, D. (2004). Perceived needs following traumatic brain injury. *Journal of Head Trauma Rehabilitation, 19*(3), 205–216.

[2] Koskinen, S. (1998). Quality of life 10 years after a very severe traumatic brain injury (TBI): The perspective of the injured and the closest relative. *Brain Injury, 12*(8), 631–648.

[3] Poggi, G., Liscio, M., Adduci, A., Galbiati, S., Sommovigo, M., Degrate, A., et al. (2003). Neuropsychiatric sequelae in TBI: A comparison across different age groups. *Brain Injury, 17*(10), 835–846.

[4] Ownsworth, T., Little, T., Turner, B., Hawkes, A., & Shum, D. (2008). Assessing emotional status following acquired brain injury: The clinical potential of the depression, anxiety and stress scales. *Brain Injury, 22*(11), 858–869.

[5] Gururaj, G., Shastry, K. V. R., Chandramouli, A. B., Subbakrishna, D. K., Kraus, J. F. (2005). *Traumatic brain injury.* National Institute of Mental Health and Neuro Sciences, Publication no. 61.

[6] Corrigan, J. D., Bogner, J. A., Mysiw, W. J., Clinchot, D., & Fugate, L. (2001). Life satisfaction after traumatic brain injury. *Journal of Head Trauma Rehabilitation, 16*(6), 543–555.

[7] Feuerstein, R., Falik, L. H., & Feuerstein, R. (1998). *Feuerstein's Instrumental Enrichment Program.* Jerusalem, Israel: International Centre for the Enhancement Potential.

[8] Griffiths, K. (1997). *"P.S. This accident has changed everyone and everything": A guide to understanding head injury.* Melbourne: Australian Psychological Society.

[9] Moore, E. L., Terryberry-Spohr, L., & Hope, D. A. (2006). Mild traumatic brain injury and anxiety sequelae: A review of the literature. *Brain Injury, 20*(2), 117–132. National Environmental Policy Act of 1969, 42 1983 (1994)

[10] Bay, E, Hagerty, B. M, Williams, R. A, Kirsch, N, & Gillespie, B. (2002). Chronic stress, sense of belonging, and depression among survivors of traumatic brain injury. *Journal of Nursing Scholarship, 34*, 221–226.

[11] Bay, E, Kirsch, N, & Gillespie, B. (2004). Chronic stress conditions do explain post-traumatic brain injury depression. *Research and Theory for Nursing Practice, 18*, 213–228.

[12] Oddy, M., Coushlan, T., Tyerman, A., & Jenkins, D. (1985). Social adjustment after closed head injury: A further follow-up seven years after injury. *Journal of Neurology, Neurosurgery and Psychiatry, 48*, 564–568.

[13] Jacobs, H. E. (1988). The Los Angeles head injury survey: Procedures and initial findings. *Archives of Physical Medicine and Rehabilitation, 69*, 425–431.

[14] Lezak, M. D., & O'Brien, K. P. (1988). Longitudinal study of emotional, social, and physical changes after traumatic brain injury. *Journal of Learning Disabilities, 21*, 456–463.

[15] Thomsen, I. V. (1984). Late outcome of very severe blunt head trauma: A 10–15 year second follow-up. *Journal of Neurology, Neurosurgery and Psychiatry, 47*, 260–268.

[16] Kaplan, S. P. (1988). Adaptation following serious brain injury: An assessment after one year. *Journal of Applied Rehabilitation Counselling, 19*(3), 3–8.

[17] Newton, A., & Johnson, D. A. (1985). Social adjustment and interaction after severe head injury. *British Journal of Clinical Psychology, 24*, 225–234.

[18] Wehman, P. H., Kreutzer, J. S., West, M. D., Sherron, P. D., Zasler, N. D., Groah, C. H., et al. (1990). Return to work for persons with traumatic brain injury: A supported employment approach. *Archives of Physical Medicine and Rehabilitation, 71*, 1047–1052.

[19] Rappaport, M., Herrero-Backe, C., Rappaport, M. L., & Winterfield, K. M. (1989). Head injury outcome up to ten years later. *Archives of Physical Medicine and Rehabilitation, 70*, 885–892.

[20] NIH Consensus Development Panel on Rehabilitation of Persons with Traumatic Brain Injury, (1999) Rehabilitation of persons with traumatic brain injury. *JAMA, 282*, 974–983.

[21] Lezak, M. D. (1995). *Neuropsychological assessment* (3rd ed.). New York: Oxford University Press.

[22] Wilson, B. A. (2009). Kate: Cognitive recovery and emotional adjustment in a young woman who was unresponsive for several months. In B. A. Wilson, F. Gracey, J. J. Evans, & A. Bateman (Eds.), *Neuropsychological rehabilitation: Theory, models, therapy and outcome* (pp. 317–333). New York: Cambridge University Press.

[23] Gracey, F., Brentnall, S., & Megoran, R. (2009). Judith: Learning to do things 'at the drop of a hat': Behavioural experiments to explore and change the 'meaning' in meaningful functional activity. In B. A. Wilson, F. Gracey, J. J. Evans, & A. Bateman (Eds.), *Neuropsychological rehabilitation: Theory, models, therapy and outcome* (pp. 256–271). New York: Cambridge University Press.

[24] Izaute, M., Durozard, C., Aldigier, E., Teissedre, F., Perreve, A, & Gerbaud, L. (2008). Perceived social support and locus of control after a traumatic brain injury (TBI). *Brain Injury, 22*(10), 758–764.

[25] Bryant, R. A, Moulds, M, Guthrie, R, & Nixon, R. D. (2003). Treating acute stress disorder following mild traumatic brain injury. *American Journal of Psychiatry, 160*, 585–587.

[26] Ozsuer, H, Gorgulu, A, Kiris, T, & Cobanoglu, S. (2005). The effects of memantine on lipid peroxidation following closed-head trauma in rats. *Neurosurgery Review, 28*, 143–147.

[27] Ratey, J. J., Leveroni, C. L., & Miller, A. C. (1992). Low-dose buspirone to treat agitation and maladaptive behavior in brain injured-patients, two case reports. *Journal of Clinical Psychopharmacology, 12,* 362–364.

[28] Fava, M. (1997). Psychopharmacologic treatment of pathologic aggression. *Psychiatry Clinical North America, 20,* 427–451.

[29] Fujii, D, & Ahmed, I. (2002). Characteristics of psychotic disorder due to traumatic brain injury: An analysis of case studies in the literature. *Journal of Neuropsychiatry and Clinical Neuroscience, 14,* 130–140.

[30] Zhang, Q., & Sachdev, P. S. (2003). Psychotic disorder and traumatic brain injury. *Current Psychiatry Reports, 5,* 197–201.

[31] Prigatano, G. P. (1988). Psychotherapy and neuropsychological assessment after brain injury. *Journal of Head Trauma Rehabilitation, 3,* 45–56.

[32] Soo, C., & Tate, R. (2007). Psychological treatment for anxiety in people with traumatic brain injury. *Cochrane Database of Systematic Reviews, 3* CD005239.

[33] Ylvisaker, M. M., Turkstra, L. M., Kennedy, M., Coelho, C., Yorkston, K. C., Sohlberg, M. M., et al. (2007). Behavioral interventions for children and adults with behavior disorders after TBI: A systematic review of the evidence. *Brain Injury, 21*(8), 769–804.

[34] Leishman, W. A. (1998). *Organic psychiatry* (3rd ed.). Oxford: Blackwell Science. 161–217.

[35] Sankla, S. K., Mishra, M., Ansman, J. I. (1998). Think first. Neuorotrauma '98. *Proceedings of Neurotrauma Conference,* Indore, 1–5.

[36] McMordie, W. R., Barker, S. L., & Paolos, T. M. (1990). Return to work (RTW) after head injury. *Brain Injury, 4,* 57–69.

[37] Ip, R. Y., Dornan, J., & Schentag, C. (1995). Traumatic brain injury: Factors predicting return to work or school. *Brain Injury, 9*(5), 517–532.

[38] Dikmen, S. S., Temkin, N. R., Machamer, J. E., Holubkov, A., Fraser, R., & Winn, R. (1994). Employment following traumatic head injuries. *Archives of Neurology, 51,* 12–24.

[39] Greenspan, A. I., Wrigley, J. M., Kresnow, M., Branche-Dorsey, C. M., & Fine, P. R. (1996). Factors influencing failure to return to work due to traumatic brain injury. *Brain Injury, 10,* 207–218.

[40] Clare, L., Wilson, B. A., Carter, G., Hodges, J. R., & Adams, M. (2001). Long-term maintenance of treatment gains following a cognitive rehabilitation intervention in early dementia of Alzheimer type: A single case study. *Cognitive Rehabilitation in Dementia: A Special Issue of Neuropsychological Rehabilitation, 11,* 477–494.

[41] Zasler, N. D., & Martelli, M. F. (2005). Sexual dysfunction. In J. M. Silver, T. W. McAllister, & S. C. Yudofsky (Eds.), *Textbook of traumatic brain injury.* Washington, DC: American Psychiatric Publishing.

[42] Kreuter, M., Dahllof, A. G., Gudjonsson, G., et al. (1998). Sexual adjustment and its predictors after traumatic brain injury. *Brain Injury, 12,* 349–368.

[43] Garden, F. H., Bontke, C. F., & Hoffman, M. (1990). Sexual functioning and marital adjustment after traumatic brain injury. *Journal of Head Trauma Rehabilitation, 5,* 52–59.

[44] Blackerby, W. (1987). Disruption of sexuality following a head injury. *National Head Injury Foundation News, 7,* 8.

[45] Miller, B, Cummings, J, McIntyre, H, Ebers, G, & Grode, M. (1986). Hypersexuality or altered sexual preference following brain injury. *Journal of Neurology & Neurosurgery Psychiatry, 49,* 867–873.

[46] Sabhesan, S., & Natarajan, M. (1989). Sexual behavior after head injury in Indian men and women. *Archives of Sexual Behavior, 18*(4), 349–356.

[47] Ponsford, J. (2003). Sexual changes associated with traumatic brain injury. *Neuropsychological Rehabilitation, 13*(1–2), 275–289.

[48] Hibbard, M. R., Gordon, W. A., Flanagan, S., Haddad, L., & Labinsky, E. (2000). Sexual dysfunction after traumatic brain injury. *Neurorehabilitation, 15*, 107–120.

[49] Mauss-Clum, N., & Ryan, M. (1981). Brain injury and the family. *Journal of Neurosurgical Nursing, 13*, 165–169.

[50] Oddy, M., & Humphrey, M. (1980). Social recovery during the first year following severe head injury. *Journal of Neurology, Neurosurgery and Psychiatry, 43*, 798–802.

[51] Lezak, M. D. (1978). Living with the characterologically altered brain injured patient. *Journal of Clinical Psychiatry, 39*, 592–598.

[52] Gosling, J., & Oddy, M. (1999). Rearranged marriages: Marital relationships after head injury. *Brain Injury, 13*(10), 785–796.

[53] Blais, M. C., & Boisvert, J-M. (2007). Psychological adjustment and marital satisfaction following head injury. Which critical personal characteristics should both partners develop? *Brain Injury, 21*(4), 357–372.

[54] Arango-Lasprilla, J. C., Ketchum, J. M., Dezfulian, T., Kreutzer, J. S., O'Neil-Pirozzi, T. M., Hammond, F., et al. (2008). Predictors of marital stability 2 years following traumatic brain injury. *Brain Injury, 22*(7–8), 565–574.

[55] Annon, J. (1976). *The behavioral treatment of sexual disorders*. Baltimore: Harper & Row.

[56] Rao, N., Rosenthal, M., Cronin-Stubbs, D., Lambert, R., Barnes, P., & Swanson, B. (1990). Return to work after rehabilitation following traumatic brain injury. *Brain Injury, 4*, 49–56.

# 4 EEG Neurofeedback Training in Clinical Conditions

## J. Rajeswaran, C.N. Bennett, S. Thomas, K. Rajakumari

Clinical Neuropsychology Unit, Department of Clinical Psychology, National Institute of Mental Health and Neurosciences (NIMHANS), Bangalore, Karnataka, India

*The real problem is not whether machines think but whether men do.*

B.F. Skinner, Contingencies of Reinforcement, 1969

Electroencephalogram (EEG) neurofeedback training (NFT) is a fairly new advance in the field of neuropsychological rehabilitation that can be formally traced back to Kamiya's work in 1963. This pioneering study [2] involved training the subject to recognize alpha activity by verbal reinforcement. Another important landmark was the incidental finding by Sterman and his colleagues of seizure resistance in cats that were trained to increase sensorimotor rhythm (SMR) [2]. The advent of NFT as a therapeutic procedure has been the source of several controversial debates. While NFT has been described as a miracle machine by some users, there are practitioners who remain skeptical. It has to be emphasized here that as in the opening quote, the vital point to be noted is that while there is significant evidence that NFT works, the method of application by a trained practitioner is of utmost importance. Neurofeedback is used to modify amplitude, frequency, and even coherency of one's own brain waves using operation conditioning methods [1]. The choice of the ideal protocol for a given patient depends, of course, on the expertise and skill of application of the therapist.

During NFT, raw signals from the brain are recorded digitally on paper or any other recordable format using EEG. Generally, neurofeedback professionals depend on the international 10–20 system. According to this system, each scalp position (19 primary sites) is assigned letters and numbers designating their location. Based on the treatment protocol, these scalp locations are used to guide placement of electrodes and relevant training is given [2].

The raw signal obtained from the EEG is further processed, analyzed, and converted into a format suitable to be used for feedback. The signal intensity or amplitude of the wave is measured in microvolts (mV) and is an important index used to

Neuropsychological Rehabilitation-Principles and Applications.
DOI: http://dx.doi.org/10.1016/B978-0-12-416046-0.00004-3

describe the wave. Another index used is the signal frequency of the wave that refers to the number of wave cycles per second. An understanding of these aspects of the waveform is important as certain activities and brain states are associated with specific types of wave patterns on the EEG.

The main frequencies of the human EEG waves are:

Delta (1–4 or 1–3.5 Hz)
Delta activity is primarily associated with sleep and is seen predominantly in infants [1]. Delta activity is normally seen during problem solving in the awake EEG. In pathological conditions, however, delta activity is suggestive of brain injury [3]. Children with attention deficit hyperactivity disorder (ADHD) or learning disorders also have abnormal activation of delta and theta bands. Reducing the delta band with the theta band may be indicated in these conditions.

Theta (4–7, 4–7.5, or 4–8 Hz)
Theta is known to be related to creativity and spontaneity. On the flip side, however, it is also associated with distractibility and other deficits of attention, daydreaming, depression, and anxiety. Normative data suggests that theta-to-beta ratios are approximately 2:1 in adults and 2.5:1 in children [2]. Any change in this pattern, particularly an increase of this activity in the anterior regions, may require protocols that reinforce its reduction.

Alpha (8–12 or 8–13 Hz)
Alpha is seen primarily in the occipital, parietal, and posterior temporal lobes. Alpha is associated with meditation and a state of relaxation. Alpha amplitudes are normally higher in posterior regions and lower in anterior regions of the brain [2].
Alpha activity usually decreases with eyes open, which is referred to as alpha blocking. Alpha is usually downregulated in the anterior side of the brain and upregulated for training for deep states of relaxation. Clinical trials have successfully used deep-state training to remediate posttraumatic stress disorder and addictions [4].

Sensorimotor rhythm (12–15 or 12–16 Hz)
SMR, sometimes referred to as low beta, is predominantly found in the sensorimotor cortex (sensorimotor strip). Ideally, SMR is found to increase when the brain's motor functions are reduced. This indicates that SMR amplitude increases with tranquillity and decreases with motility [2]. Barry Sterman and his colleagues are well known for their work with SMR training. Hyperactive clients with decreased levels of SMR are likely to improve with uptraining at Cz or C4 [2].

Beta (13–21 Hz)
Increased beta activity in the left frontal cortex is a marker for depression, and decreased activity in the right frontal cortex is a marker for anxiety [2]. This indicates that upregulating the left hemisphere anterior beta may be indicated for depression, whereas downregulating right hemisphere anterior beta may be useful in treating anxiety.

EEG training systems include both single-channel as well as two-channel systems. Two-channel training systems are generally preferred as they are more versatile and can train two scalp locations simultaneously while comparing them. Two-channel protocols include coherence training, phase training, alpha synchrony, rectifying asymmetries, as well as training along the sensorimotor cortex.

EEG NFT has been used in various clinical conditions as a primary treatment or as an adjunct treatment. It is well known that human activity is dependent on the flow of information through elaborate neuronal networks in the brain. Different activities and functions are associated with different brainwaves. A healthy brain shifts through different brainwave states depending on the task the individual has to address, whereas in a disregulated brain, there may be underarousal, unresponsiveness, or overarousal, resulting in difficulty responding adequately to environmental demands. EEG neurofeedback addresses these difficulties by enhancing the brain function, thereby improving the brain's ability to switch states. In other words, the brain regulates overall health and performance. Importantly, NFT taps into the natural mechanisms that make a brain learn, grow, and heal itself. Research in EEG neurofeedback has documented its value in the treatment of several clinical conditions. It is noninvasive, holistic, and there are no significant negative side effects. It resolves problems instead of temporarily suppressing them. The patient's own internal systems develop the ability to perform well on their own, without having to depend on drugs.

EEG NFT has found wide application in various clinical syndromes, such as migraine [5,6], tinnitus [7–9], stroke [10], depression [11,12], epilepsy [13,14], obsessive–compulsive disorder [15], and ADHD [16,17].

The following sections attempt to discuss the effectiveness of NFT in alcohol dependence syndrome (ADS), traumatic brain injury (TBI), and stroke.

## Alcohol Dependence Syndrome

According to the World Health Organization (WHO), there are approximately 2 billion people worldwide who consume alcoholic beverages and 76.3 million with diagnosable alcohol use disorders [18]. The global burden related to alcohol consumption, in terms of both morbidity and mortality, is considerable and is fast becoming a major source of concern for most countries in the world. Alcohol addiction can be a dangerous preoccupation, leading to severe mental as well as physical problems. Uncontrolled alcohol consumption over a long period of time may result in withdrawal tendencies and dependence, often inescapable and damaging. Addiction to alcohol has been identified by the WHO as a mental/behavioral disorder warranting treatment [19], characterized by physiological and psychological signs of dependence, which include craving, loss of control, withdrawal, tolerance, salience, and use of alcohol despite evidence and knowledge of harmful effects of alcohol. The various problems arising from alcohol abuse affect social, financial, occupational, and cognitive domains. India, which is considered a relatively dry country, has a prevalence rate of 21% [20]. The problem of alcoholism poses a major problem, especially in India, due to the susceptibility to dependence and also due to the fact that a vast majority of the individuals who are addicted to alcohol are the primary bread winners of the family. Alcoholism is considered to derive from both genetic and social causes. As with all psychiatric disorders, a genetic predisposition interacts with environmental factors to heighten vulnerability to produce the illness.

## Cognitive Impairment in ADS

Alcohol can induce a wide spectrum of effects on the central nervous system. These effects can be recognized at the neurochemical, neurophysiological, neuroanatomical, and neuropsychological levels. Researchers have used a variety of techniques and have concluded that patients who use alcohol have effects on the frontal lobes, the limbic system, and the cerebellum [21–24].

The relationship between abstinence and recovery of deficits in chronic alcoholics is only partly understood. The most severe impairments may partially resolve in the initial 1–4 weeks following cessation of drinking; however, recovery processes may extend over the course of a year or more. Verbal functions are the first to recover, whereas memory and visuospatial skills recover very slowly. Deficits may continue to be present in new learning and complex or novel problem solving [25]. Alcohol-dependent individuals tend to have deficits in executive functions, which may lead to relapse [26], because the patient may not be able to use information regarding treatment and rehabilitation given immediately after cessation of drinking until the deficits are resolved [27]. Recovery is also dependent on abstinence and other comorbid conditions.

Alcohol-dependent individuals are found to have low levels of alpha and theta waves and a greater amount of fast beta brain waves in their EEGs [28]. This makes it inherently difficult for them to relax. Consuming alcohol helps to increase the alpha and theta waves. Alcohol-dependent individuals thus are treating themselves using an agent that helps them to relax, and this state of relaxation is highly reinforcing for them [29]. Several studies have shown that training alcohol-dependent individuals to increase their alpha and theta rhythms is associated with a decrease in alcohol intake and prevents relapse [30,31]. EEG alpha and theta oscillations are shown to represent cognitive and memory performance [32]. Studies have shown that increasing alpha power can increase cognitive functions in normal individuals [33]. Information transfer and integration in the brain that leads to high-level cognitive processes requires neuronal coordination. Alpha waves in EEG activity are considered to aid the integration of cognition [34].

Several studies have shown that neurofeedback is effective in treating and preventing relapse in alcohol-dependent individuals. Peniston and Kulkosky were the pioneers in this field. Most studies have used alpha and theta brain wave training. They show that NFT is useful in the rehabilitation of alcoholics. Most studies have used outcome measures that include anxiety and depression scores, personality dimensions, relapse rate, and coping. In treatment of alcoholics, the number of sessions ranges from 20 to 50 [35]. Only one study has taken into account cognitive variables like attention [36].

A study [37] was undertaken to study the efficacy of NFT in alcohol-dependent individuals. The sample included 40 patients who fulfilled the criteria for ICD 10 (F 10.2) diagnosis of ADS. They were recruited from inpatients of the Deaddiction Unit, Department of Psychiatry, NIMHANS, Bangalore, after obtaining informed consent. The study was conducted in three stages: pretraining assessment, the NFT, and posttraining assessment. A baseline of the EEG on two channels on the neurofeedback machine was done for all the patients. The treatment group received NFT along with routine treatment and medication in the ward, and the treatment-as-usual group received only the routine treatment and medication in the ward. Treatment as usual led to improvement in cognitive functions. The addition of NFT led to further improvement in quality of life (QOL), cognitive functions, and reduced relapse rates at 1-month follow-up.

---

### Case Vignette

Mr. K, a 29-year-old married male, educated up to seventh standard, from low socioeconomic background, working as an agricultural laborer, was admitted for the second time with a history of drinking alcohol for the past 15 years. He first used alcohol when he was 14 years of age, and started drinking daily at the age of 19 years. The patient had developed symptoms of withdrawal, tolerance, craving, loss of control, and was using alcohol despite the knowledge of harmful effects. Prior to admission in the hospital, patient was drinking about 720 ml of brandy in a day. The patient had been married for the past 7 years, and had no children. The patient's alcohol-related problems led to marital discord, and the patient and his wife were living separately. The patient was very irregular at work and would spend most of his earnings on drinking. The patient's wife was working in a garment factory and had to take care of the family. They had arguments every day, as the patient wanted money from the wife to drink, which would end in violent behavior, including assaulting the wife on many occasion. The wife had decided not to have children as she realized that the children would only add to her burden. The patient was not motivated to give up drinking and had got admitted due to external pressure from the wife and other members of the family. The patient was admitted earlier and had relapsed on the same day of discharge and was constantly threatening that he would start drinking as soon as he was discharged. The patient was admitted to the special ward, as the patient's wife believed that other patients in the general ward would influence the patient to drink after discharge.

The patient was recruited for the study three days after admission to the ward. It was very difficult to establish rapport with the patient, and the motivation to undergo treatment was poor. However, the patient agreed to participate in the study as he had no other activity after the scheduled group therapy and individual sessions. During the initial assessment, patient rapport could not be established, though he would answer the questions asked. However, he was motivated to undergo the neuropsychological assessment as the patient found the tests interesting. The NFT sessions started immediately after the neuropsychological assessment. The patient would not keep appointments for the initial sessions and had to be personally contacted for each session. He also had difficulty in understanding the concept of operant conditioning and the reward points that he received as a result of relaxation through NFT.

*Procedure*: NFT was carried out in a quiet, dimly lit room. The patient was seated on a comfortable chair in front of the neurofeedback machine. The desired electrode positions (i.e., O1 and O2) were noted and the hair was parted, exposing the scalp over the desired locations. The scalp was cleaned and prepared with an abrasive gel, scrubbing lightly to clean the skin surface. A pea-sized ball of 10–20 paste was applied to the cup of the gold electrodes, taking care not to stress the electrode mounting collar. The electrode was pressed onto the scalp using a cotton ball to press it down and ensure a secure connection to the skin. The ear lobes were cleaned using abrasive gel, using the thumb and forefinger to scrub the skin. A pea-sized ball of 10–20 paste was scooped into each cup of the ear clip. The ear clips were clipped to lobes of both ears. The reference electrode was also connected to the Cz position in the aforementioned procedure. The wires from the sensors were plugged into the connectors on the front of the neurofeedback machine, using the appropriate colors for each lead. The program was then turned on. The protocol was selected (i.e., the alpha theta training for relaxation). The procedure and the goals were explained to the patient thoroughly before starting the session, and the nature of the task was also explained. The display screen was then selected. With the screen on, it was again explained to the patient what the rewards were and how to increase the points. The rewards were given through visual feedback, auditory feedback, and an increase in the score displayed on the screen. Twenty sessions of NFT were conducted. Each session was of 40-min duration, with a minimum of four sessions per week. After the first 5–6 sessions, the patient's motivation was found to be better when he realized that he could control the task and the reward points that he obtained in the NFT, after which he was punctual for the sessions; by the third week, he was able to relax and increase the reward points. He was also found to be interested in the postassessment that was carried out before the patients' discharge.

The patient was given a follow-up date after a month, and the patient and his wife came for the follow-up assessment. The patient had maintained abstinence for the month and had also started going for work regularly for the first time in several years, as reported by his wife. Incidences of arguments at home had decreased. The couple was again followed up at 2 and 3 months, and the patient continued to maintain abstinence and treatment gains at 3 months.

The results indicate improvement on psychosocial and neuropsychological variables postintervention (Figures 4.1 and 4.2). NFT has been found effective in the treatment of ADS. Alpha theta training has been found to be effective in improving clinical symptoms of depression and anxiety, changing personality patterns, and preventing relapse in alcohol-dependent individuals.

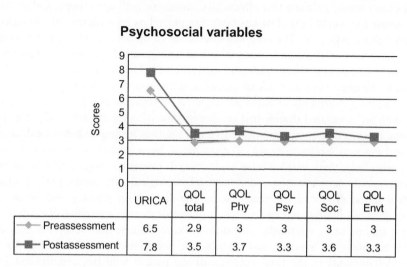

**Figure 4.1  Comparison of the psychosocial variables pre- and post-NFT.** URICA, University of Rhode Island Change Assessment Scale; QOL, Quality of Life; Phy, Physical; Psy, Psychological; Soc, Social; Envt, Environment.

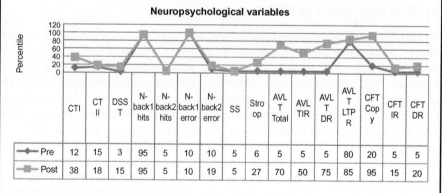

**Figure 4.2  Comparison of neuropsychological variables pre- and post-NFT.** CT, Color Trails; DSST, Digit Symbol Substitution Test; SS, Spatial Span; AVLT, Auditory Verbal Learning Test; CFT, Complex Figure Test; IR, Immediate Recall; DR, Delayed Recall; LTPR, Long-Term Percent Retention.

# Traumatic Brain Injury

According to WHO, TBI will be the major cause of death and disability by the year 2020. There are an estimated 10 million people affected annually by TBI, due to which the burden of mortality and morbidity is increasing [38]. TBI is a major health and socioeconomic problem that affects all communities, all age groups, and all societies across the world [39]. TBI has been recognized as an affliction of humankind since the Stone Age [40]. The complex interaction of human, vehicle, environmental factors, and the use of alcohol, along with a lack of sustainable preventive programs, has contributed to the "silent epidemic" of TBIs [41]. TBI is considered an insult or trauma to the brain from an external mechanical force, possibly leading to temporary or permanent impairments of physical, cognitive, emotional, and psychosocial functions with an associated diminished or altered state of consciousness [42]. TBI is a dynamic process that involves damage to the brain, thus leading to behavioral, cognitive, and emotional consequences. At the time of head trauma, a series of destructive intracellular and extracellular pathological processes begin, which include neurochemical, neuroanatomic, and neurophysiological alterations [43]. Damage to brain tissue produced by head trauma results in both primary and secondary effects. Primary injuries are caused by a number of events, including direct trauma, indirect trauma (e.g., whiplash), and diffuse axonal injury. Secondary brain insults include hypotension, hypoxia, and anemia. The degree and type of brain insults are major determinants in the final outcome of the patient who has experienced TBI. Preexisting factors, such as the patient's age and trauma-related systemic events, also impact brain insult [44]. TBI has a series of physical and mental symptoms. The bio-socio-occupational dysfunction experienced by the patients leads to poor QOL [45].

## Cognitive Impairment in TBI

TBI survivors experience persistent cognitive deficits in attention, concentration, and memory. Studies indicate impaired ability to focus attention [46], deficits in selective, divided, and sustained attentions [47–49]. Patients commonly report becoming excessively forgetful and slower in performing complex mental activities. Deficits in the speed of information processing have also been reported [50,51]. Impairment in higher-level executive functions such as reasoning, planning, problem solving, emotional self-regulation, and judgment is indicated [52]. Memory impairment has been frequently reported in TBI cases [53–56]. Neuropsychological deficits are found to vary with the severity of TBI. Temkin et al. [55] found an association between head injury severity and scores on measures of verbal learning and memory and information processing speed at 3–5 years post injury. Similarly, they found a relationship between patients' performance on memory and a measure of long-term functional status. Hanks et al. [57] found that measures of verbal memory and executive functions/processing speed were related to measures of functional outcome 6 months after acute rehabilitation. These studies have examined and evaluated the relationship between injury severity and neurocognitive impairment, as well as the relative contribution of these parameters to functional outcome, thereby resulting in poor QOL.

Young Indian males in the productive stage of life tend to suffer these consequences of brain damage, disrupting the family functioning. As cognitive impairments are the most persistent and prominent sequelae of brain injury in patients with TBI, the need for neuropsychological evaluation and retraining emerges. Comprehensive neuropsychological rehabilitation seeks to retrain and reeducate patients with disabling injuries to compromise or cope with existing problems and to improve levels of daily functioning [58].

## Neurofeedback Training in TBI

NFT was carried out in TBI first by Ayers [59], who used alpha quantitative electro-encephalograph (QEEG) training in 250 cases and demonstrated return to premorbid functioning in a significant number of cases. Thatcher et al. [60] used QEEG to distinguish between 608 adult patients with Mild Traumatic Brain Injury (MTBI) and 108 age-matched controls. Measures included anterior–posterior amplitude gradients, posterior relative power, and the interelectrode comparison measurements of phase and coherence in the frontal and temporal lobes. Initial analysis of 264 patients and 83 normals proved that the QEEG method was successful in distinguishing the mild TBI group from the control group, achieving an overall discriminant classification accuracy of 94.8%. The MTBI group exhibited neurophysiological features such as increased coherence and decreased phases in frontal and frontotemporal regions, reduced alpha band amplitudes in the parieto-occipital regions, and decreased power difference between anterior/posterior cortical regions. Peniston et al. [61] later reported improved symptoms in Vietnam veterans with combat-related posttraumatic disorders who used neurofeedback. Hoffman et al. [62] reported 80% of mildly posttraumatic head-injured patients who demonstrated improvements in self-reported symptoms and neuropsychological measures after an average of 40 sessions of NFT. Rozelle and Budzynski [63] gave audio/visual stimulation and 48 sessions NFT to a 55-year-old male who had suffered a left posterior temporal/parietal cerebrovascular accident post-1 year. The patient was trained to decrease slower 4–7 Hz theta waves and increase faster 15–21 Hz activity over sensorimotor and speech areas. He demonstrated significant pre- versus posttraining changes on neuropsychological tests assessing aphasia, on a self-report inventory of psychological distress, and from an independent speech evaluation. Hoffman et al. [64] reported that 80% of mildly posttraumatic head-injury patients demonstrate improvements in self-reported symptoms and neuropsychological measures after an average of 40 sessions of NFT. A similar finding reported by Ham and Packard [65] evaluated NFT in 40 individuals with posttraumatic head injury and found reduction of symptoms by 53% and 80% improvement in the ability to relax. Thornton [66] compared three patients with post-head injury and reported 68–81% improvement in mean recall of paragraphs after amplitude and coherence NFT. He created a normative QEEG database that assessed correlates of effective memory functioning. He compared three patients (two post-head injury and one post-hippocampal surgery) QEEGs during paragraph recall to the database and devised individualized treatment protocols to remediate their deficits. He reported that his three patients demonstrated 68–81% improvement in the mean recall of paragraphs post-NFT. Keller [67] evaluated NFT in remediation of attention deficits in patients with moderate Closed Head Injury (CHI). Feedback of beta activity (13–20 Hz) was used for 12 patients. A matched control group of nine patients was treated with a standard computerized training (speed of information processing and selective attention). Feedback concerning speed and accuracy was immediately provided by the microcomputer during the task. Training sessions of 10–30 min were conducted over 2 weeks for normal control. All patients were tested before and after treatment with a set of attention tests (letter cancellation, simple choice reaction, and sustained attention task). Results indicated that after 10 sessions the analyses of beta activity showed that 8 patients were able to increase their beta activity while the remaining 4 patients showed a decrease of beta activity. Mean duration of beta activity was prolonged about 50% after training. Patients who received NFT improved significantly more in the attention tests than control patients. Zelek [68] examined NFT in patients with acquired brain injury. Ten patients with moderate to severe brain injury participated in the study. Cognitive abilities were assessed with the repeatable battery for the assessment of neuropsychological status (RBANS) pre- and post-NFT. NFT was given 2–3 times a week for the total of 30 sessions. Results indicated that in all 10 patients, RBANS measures were found to be significantly improved following NFT. All subjects showed significant improvement in their brainwave power and coherence values. Reddy et al. [56] examined NFT used to enhance verbal and visual learning and memory in a patient with TBI. A single case study design was adopted. The neuropsychological profile of the patient was compared pre- and post-NFT. Patient S, a 30-year-old male with mild head injury, was given sessions of NFT, 45 min/day, 5 days a week. The training incorporated video feedback to increase the frequency of alpha waves (8–12 Hz) and to decrease theta waves (4–7 Hz). The preassessment showed impairment in verbal learning and memory. Results indicated improvement in both verbal and visual learning memory in the patient post-NFT.

Studies in the field of NFT indicate that it can be used to enhance cognitive functions. TBI has adverse effects on cognitive, emotional, and behavioral functioning. Cognitive rehabilitation has been found to be effective in treating these deficits. There are a number of techniques which are emerging to ameliorate these deficits. The use of NFT is increasing in rehabilitating patients. Trauma is the leading cause of long-term disability in young persons in their productive years. They present with physical, cognitive, emotional, and social disabilities depending on the severity of TBI. This inflicts burdens not only on the family but also on the country at large. This imposes greater responsibilities and requires better treatment from healthcare professionals. Newer, simpler methods and time- and cost-effective techniques should be developed in order to reach all strata of the society.

In TBI, impairments in cognitive functions have a bearing on biopsychosocial and occupational functioning. Remediation of these functions is carried out through neuropsychological rehabilitation. NFT has been effective in patients with TBI. Studies have shown improvement in patients with as few as 2 to approximately 40 sessions. As patients have shown improvement in biopsychosocial function, this form of training is cost- and time-effective and not labor intensive. In the Indian setting, there is a paucity of published studies using NFT in clinical conditions. A study was conducted at NIMHANS researching NFT in TBI. The neuropsychological assessment was carried out for right-handed patients [69]. The sample comprised 60 patients, 30 each in the intervention group (IG) and wait-list group (WG). There was a significant difference between the groups on sociodemographic and clinical details (number of years of education, rural versus urban background, severity, and assessment period). Patients in IG underwent neuropsychological assessment [70] post-1 year of TBI. The mean number of years in IG was greater than WG. With respect to background, a majority of IG were from urban environments, as opposed to rural in the WG. The neuropsychological profile of patients with TBI showed significant impairment in the speed of information processing and verbal learning and memory. The two groups were comparable at pretraining assessment except for verbal memory. There was a negative correlation of postconcussive symptoms [71,72] with QOL [73]. Positive correlation was found between neuropsychological functioning and QOL. Age and education were positively and negatively correlated with some aspect of symptoms and neuropsychological functioning. There was improvement in both groups in the postassessment, but the improvement in the IG was significant compared to WG. Postconcussion symptoms improved significantly in both IG and WG. QOL improved significantly in the IG compared to WG. There was no statistical significant improvement in the EEG post-NFT. However, on inspection there was alpha enhancement and theta inhibition. The distribution of gender and severity of injury was not equal in the two groups. Pre- and post-EEG were not recorded for WG. The study did not use a random method of sampling. Follow-up could not be carried out for all the patients (Rajakumari et al., unpublished Ph.D. thesis).

---

### Case Vignette

Mr. M, a 32-year-old married male, educated up to tenth standard, from lower socioeconomic status, suburban background, was working as a garment supervisor. He met with a road traffic accident 8 months prior to reporting to NIMHANS. He was diagnosed with severe TBI. His CT scan revealed frontotemporal involvement. He reported weakness of the right upper limb, memory loss, aggressiveness, and sleeplessness. He had well-adjusted premorbid level of functioning. Patient had good family support.

*Procedure:* NFT was carried out in a quiet, dimly lit room. The patient was seated on a comfortable chair in front of the neurofeedback machine. The desired electrode positions (O1 and O2) were marked. The protocol selected was alpha theta training for relaxation. The procedure and the goals were explained to the patient thoroughly before starting the session, and the nature of the task was also explained. The display screen was then selected. With the screen on, it was again explained to the patient as to what the rewards were and how to increase the points. The rewards were given through visual feedback, auditory feedback, and an increase in the score displayed on the screen. Twenty sessions of NFT were conducted. Each session was of 40-min duration, with a minimum of four sessions per week. Patient showed significant improvement on postconcussion symptoms, QOL, and neuropsychological variables (Figures 4.3–4.5).

Pre-NFT assessment indicated the neuropsychological profile had deficits in all domains, except for digit vigilance and visuoconstructive ability. All the pretest scores were under the 15th percentile. His profile indicated involvement of the frontotemporal lobe. He was given 20 sessions, following which a post-neuropsychological assessment was carried out. The postassessment indicates that the patient moved from the deficit range to the no-deficit range across all domains except for right-hand motor speed (Figure 4.5).

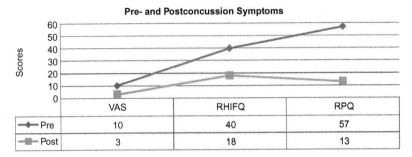

**Pre- and Postconcussion Symptoms**

| | VAS | RHIFQ | RPQ |
|---|---|---|---|
| Pre | 10 | 40 | 57 |
| Post | 3 | 18 | 13 |

**Figure 4.3 Comparison of pre- and postconcussion symptoms.** RHIFQ, Rivermead Head Injury Follow-up Questionnaire; RPQ, Rivermead Postconcussion Questionnaire; VAS, Visual analog Scale.

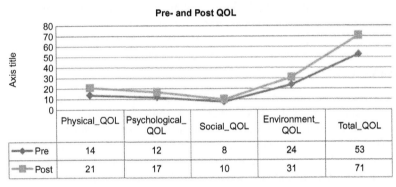

**Pre- and Post QOL**

| | Physical_QOL | Psychological_QOL | Social_QOL | Environment_QOL | Total_QOL |
|---|---|---|---|---|---|
| Pre | 14 | 12 | 8 | 24 | 53 |
| Post | 21 | 17 | 10 | 31 | 71 |

**Figure 4.4 Comparison of pre- and post-QOL.** QOL Phy, QOL physical; QOL Psy, QOL psychological; QOL Soc, QOL social; QOL Envn, QOL environment.

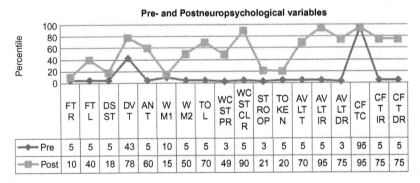

**Pre- and Postneuropsychological variables**

| | FT R | FT L | DS ST | DV T | AN T | W M1 | W M2 | TO L | WC ST PR | WC ST CL R | ST RO OP | TO KE N | AV LT T | AV LT IR | AV LT DR | CF TC | CF T IR | CF T DR |
|---|---|---|---|---|---|---|---|---|---|---|---|---|---|---|---|---|---|---|
| Pre | 5 | 5 | 5 | 43 | 5 | 10 | 5 | 5 | 3 | 5 | 3 | 5 | 5 | 5 | 3 | 95 | 5 | 5 |
| Post | 10 | 40 | 18 | 78 | 60 | 15 | 50 | 70 | 49 | 90 | 21 | 20 | 70 | 95 | 75 | 95 | 75 | 75 |

**Figure 4.5 Pre- and postneuropsychological assessment.** FTR, Finger Tapping Test (Right), FTL, Finger Tapping Test (Left); DSST, Digit Symbol Substitution Test; DVT, Digit Vigilance Test; ANT, Animal Names Test; WM 1 B H, Working Memory 1 Back Hits; WM 2 B H, Working Memory 2 Back Hits; TOL, Tower of London Test; WCST PR, Wisconsin Card Sorting test (Perseverative Responses); WCST CLR, Wisconsin Card Sorting test (Conceptual Level Responses); STROOP, Stroop Test; AVLT, Auditory Verbal Learning Test (IR: Immediate Recall, DR, Delayed Recall); CFT, Complex Figure Test (IR, Immediate Recall; DR, Delayed Recall).

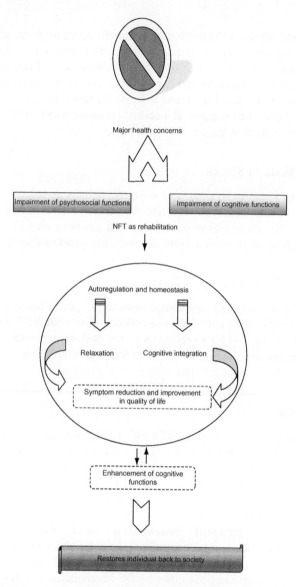

**Figure 4.6** Mechanism of the NFT as a rehabilitation for ADS and TBI.

In summary, NFT is effective in ameliorating deficits in cognitive functions and QOL in patients with TBI. Improvements were corroborated by the clinical interview with patients and significant others post-NFT. As TBI is on the rise in India, this study has demonstrated that NFT is effective in ameliorating cognitive functions and QOL in patients with TBI. It is cost- and time-effective and less labor intensive (Figure 4.6).

# Stroke

Across the world, stroke is the third most common source of death, after only coronary heart disease and cancer. In India, these statistics are altered, with stroke being the most common cause of death 2006 [76]. The prevalence of cerebrovascular disorders in India is approximately 150 per 100,000 2004 [77]. While death rates from cardiovascular diseases have been found to be on the downslide, the fact remains that the burden of disease still remains. Rehabilitation of survivors then becomes a vital aspect of future research in stroke.

## Cognitive Deficits in Stroke

There have been found to be significant cognitive deficits associated with peripheral vascular disease, including those of attention, executive functions, and visuospatial abilities 1997 [78]. Poststroke depression as well has been found to be highly correlated with deficits of problem solving, memory, and psychomotor speed 1999 [79].

## EEG Neurofeedback Training in Stroke

Rozelle and Budzynski [63] report improvement of speech fluency, word finding, balance and coordination, attention, and concentration with NFT used to increase 15–21 Hz and inhibit 4–7 Hz over sensorimotor and speech areas. Symptoms of depression, anxiety, and tinnitus as well were found to be reduced.

---

### Case Vignette

The participant was a 58-year-old male, college-educated, from an upper-middle-class socioeconomic status. The patient had been premorbidly high functioning prior to the occurrence of stroke. Primary complaints included memory loss, right-side weakness, blurred vision, and the inability to distinguish the color yellow. Assessments of cognitive deficits were made before and after 40 sessions of EEG NFT.

*Procedure*: An informed consent was taken from the participant. Preassessment included assessment of cognitive deficits, baseline EEG recordings of theta, alpha, lobeta, and beta amplitude averages taken as recorded on the O1 and O2 scalp locations given by the International 10–20 system in the first EEG neurofeedback session. A visual analog scale of symptom severity was rated by the patient and his wife.

The NIMHANS neuropsychology battery was used to assess cognitive deficits [70]. The finger tapping test was used to assess motor speed [80] and the animal names test for category fluency. A verbal n-back test was administered to assess verbal working memory. The Tower of London test was used to assess

---

planning. Performance was assessed on time taken to reach the end state and the number of moves taken to achieve it. The Wisconsin Card Sorting test was used to assess concept formation, set shifting, and maintenance of set, the Stroop test to assess response inhibition, and the token test for verbal comprehension. Rey's Auditory Verbal Learning test was used to assess verbal learning and memory, and a complex figure test to assess visuospatial construction, visual learning, and memory. The Bender Gestalt test consists of nine designs and is used to assess visuospatial construction using the principle of the perceptual tendency to organize things into a whole (Gestalt). Focal signs assessed include finger agnosia, visual object agnosia, tactile agnosia, ideational apraxia, ideomotor apraxia, dressing apraxia, construction apraxia, body schema disturbances, route finding difficulty, acalculia, and agraphia.

*Intervention*: The patient was administered 40 sessions of EEG NFT. The protocol for training was beta lobeta training at the O1 and O2 scalp locations, as described by the International 10–20 system.

*Results and Discussion*: Preassessment of cognitive deficits on the NIMHANS neuropsychology battery indicated deficits in motor speed (left hand), category fluency, planning of complex tasks, concept formation, set shifting, response inhibition, and verbal comprehension of complex instructions. Planning of simple tasks, verbal working memory, verbal learning and memory, and visual memory and visuospatial construction were found to be adequate. On the visual analog scale, the patient and his wife reported extreme visual loss, decrease in speech fluency, increased anxiety, and decreased memory. Patient continued to take physiotherapy for his motor deficits during the course of the EEG NFT.

Results indicate improvement in cognitive functions such as left motor speed, category fluency, concept formation, set shifting, response inhibition, verbal comprehension, immediate and delayed verbal memory, verbal recognition, immediate and delayed visual retention, and visuospatial construction (Figure 4.7). Normalization was defined as a shift of percentile from the deficit range to the normal range; improvement was defined as shift of percentile to a higher level by more than one quartile; and decline was defined as a shift of percentile to a lower level by more than one quartile.

Speech fluency has been known to decline with obstructive stroke (Lezak, 1995 [81]). However, the patient showed improvement on category fluency. The Wisconsin Card Sorting test is used to assess one's ability to form concepts and shift them when required, as stipulated by a changing environment. This test also assesses one's mode of learning (i.e., trial and error learning or insightful learning). Research indicates that impaired performance on The Wisconsin Card Sorting test is associated with dorsolateral prefrontal cortex impairment. Post-NFT assessment indicates

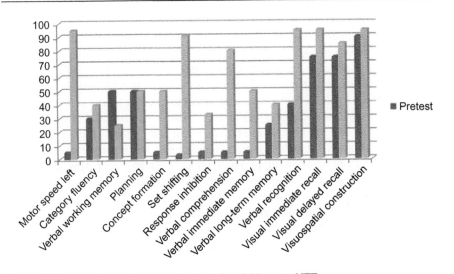

**Figure 4.7** Comparison of neuropsychological variables post-NFT.

that patients have significantly improved in terms of ability to form concepts as well as ability to shift sets where required.

Response inhibition refers to one's ability to suppress a habitual response in favor of an unusual one depending on the changing needs of the environment. Response inhibition was assessed using the Stroop Color Word test. Lesion studies implicate bilateral superior medial prefrontal damage in impaired performance on the Stroop test. Results indicate significant improvement in response inhibition posttraining.

Verbal learning includes recent memory and learning capacity and looks at efficiency in retaining newly learned information. Verbal memory looks at both immediate retention and long-held information and its retrieval, also known as remote memory. Individuals with left temporal lesions perform significantly worse than those with right temporal lesions. Assessment of visual memory requires a visuomotor response generally, and the complex figure test assesses both immediate and delayed recalls. Patients who have right hemispheric damage tend to lose several details of the figure (Lezak, 1995 [81]). The patient has shown improvement on both verbal and visual immediate and delayed recall. Visuospatial construction as well was found to be improved on the complex figure test.

EEG recordings indicate increases in amplitude of lobeta, beta, alpha, and theta, which peak and then decrease in amplitude to baseline performance. Thus, it appears that electrophysiological changes are nonpermanent and the improvement in cognition and symptom reduction may involve pathways that may not necessarily be restricted to an electrophysiological one (Figure 4.8).

Vision was reported to have improved after training by a renowned ophthalmologist. As this was an incidental and unexpected finding, no formal pre- and post-assessment of vision was undertaken (Figure 4.9).

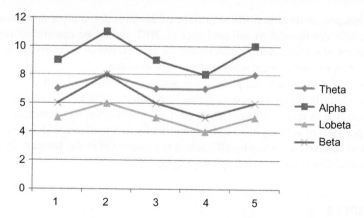

**Figure 4.8** Comparison of amplitudes of waves theta, alpha, lobeta and beta across 40 sessions of EEG NFT.

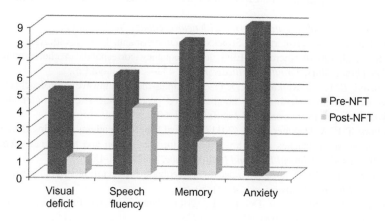

**Figure 4.9** Comparison of findings on visual analog scale post-NFT.

## Conclusion

NFT is sometimes understood as a machine–human interface. The role of the therapist, however, should never be underestimated. NFT has its value only in the context of a holistic treatment of the patient, which requires sensitivity on the part of a trained therapist. ADS, TBI, and stroke are three major health concerns contributing to both psychosocial and cognitive impairment. Evidence shows that NFT is a mechanism capable of overcoming these impairments. NFT uses autoregulation to maintain homeostasis, which helps in improving the psychosocial and cognitive functions using relaxation and cognitive integration. NFT, when used as rehabilitation, aids in recovery, which in turn restores the individual to his/her optimal level of functioning.

NFT has proven its effectiveness in three of the most debilitating problems which are extremely detrimental to self and society. NFT should be researched further in other clinical conditions and to understand the mechanism of recovery; however, its implication in routine clinical services cannot be doubted.

Duffy [74], a professor and pediatric neurologist at Harvard Medical School, has said that scholarly literature now suggests that neurofeedback "should play a major therapeutic role in many different areas … if any medication has demonstrated such a wide spectrum of efficacy it would be universally accepted and widely used … . It is a field to be taken seriously by all", stated in an editorial in the January, 2000 issue of the journal Clinical Electroencephalography.

# References

[1] Thatcher, R. W., Moore, N., John, E. R., Duffy, F., Hughes, J. R., & Krieger, M. (1999). QEEG and traumatic brain injury: Rebuttal of the American Academy of Neurology 1997 report by the EEG and clinical neuroscience society. *Clinical Electroencephalography*, *30*(3), 94–98.

[2] Demos, J. N. (2005). *Getting started with neurofeedback*. W.W. Norton.

[3] Gavilanes, A. W., Gantert, M., Strackx, E., Zimmermann, L. J., Seeldrayers, S., Vles, J. S., et al. (2010). Increased EEG delta frequency corresponds to chorioamnionitis-related brain injury. *Frontiers in Bioscience*, *2*, 432–438. (School Ed).

[4] Peniston, E. G., & Kulkosky, P. J. (1991). Alpha–theta brainwave neurofeedback therapy for Vietnam veterans with combat-related posttraumatic stress disorder. *Medical Psychotherapy. An International Journal*, *4*, 47–60.

[5] Collura, T. F., & Thatcher, R. W. (2011). Clinical benefit to patients suffering from recurrent migraine headaches and who opted to stop medication and take a neurofeedback treatment series. *Clinical EEG and Neuroscience*, *42*(2), VIII–IX.

[6] Walker, J. E. (2011). QEEG-guided neurofeedback for recurrent migraine headaches. *Clinical EEG and Neuroscience*, *42*(1), 59–61.

[7] Crocetti, A., Forti, S., & Del Bo, L. (2011). Neurofeedback for subjective tinnitus patients. *Auris Nasus Larynx*, *38*(6), 735–738.

[8] Schenk, S., Lamm, K., Gundel, H., & Ladwig, K. H. (2005). [Neurofeedback-based EEG alpha and EEG beta training. Effectiveness in patients with chronically decompensated tinnitus]. *HNO*, *53*(1), 29–37.

[9] Gosepath, K., Nafe, B., Ziegler, E., & Mann, W. J. (2001). [Neurofeedback in therapy of tinnitus]. *HNO*, *49*(1), 29–35.

[10] Wing, K. (2001). Effect of neurofeedback on motor recovery of a patient with brain injury: A case study and its implications for stroke rehabilitation. *Topics in Stroke Rehabilitation*, *8*(3), 45–53.

[11] Choi, S. W., Chi, S. E., Chung, S. Y., Kim, J. W., Ahn, C. Y., & Kim, H. T. (2011). Is alpha wave neurofeedback effective with randomized clinical trials in depression? A pilot study. *Neuropsychobiology*, *63*(1), 43–51.

[12] Dias, A. M., & van Deusen, A. (2011). A new neurofeedback protocol for depression. *The Spanish Journal of Psychology*, *14*(1), 374–384.

[13] Walker, J. E. (2008). Power spectral frequency and coherence abnormalities in patients with intractable epilepsy and their usefulness in long-term remediation of seizures using neurofeedback. *Clinical EEG and Neuroscience*, *39*(4), 203–205.

[14] Sterman, M. B., & Egner, T. (2006). Foundation and practice of neurofeedback for the treatment of epilepsy. *Applied Psychophysiology and Biofeedback, 31*(1), 21–35.

[15] Surmeli, T., & Ertem, A. (2011). Obsessive compulsive disorder and the efficacy of qEEG-guided neurofeedback treatment: A case series. *Clinical EEG and Neuroscience, 42*(3), 195–201.

[16] Drechsler, R., Straub, M., Doehnert, M., Heinrich, H., Steinhausen, H. C., & Brandeis, D. (2007). 1Controlled evaluation of a neurofeedback training of slow cortical potentials in children with Attention Deficit/Hyperactivity Disorder (ADHD). *Behavioral and Brain Functions, 3*, 35.

[17] Butnik, S. M. (2005). Neurofeedback in adolescents and adults with attention deficit hyperactivity disorder. *Journal of Clinical Psychology, 61*(5), 621–625.

[18] The World Health Report, (2002). *Reducing risks, promoting healthy life.* Geneva: WHO.

[19] World Health Organization, (1992). *The ICD 10 classification of mental and behavioural disorders.* Geneva: WHO.

[20] Ray, R., Mondal, A. B., Gupta, K., Chatterjee, A., & Bajaj, P. (2004). *The extent, pattern and trends of drug abuse in India: National survey.* New Delhi: United Nations Office on Drugs and Crimes and Ministry of Social Justice and Empowerment, Government of India.

[21] Moselhy, H. F., Georgiou, G., & Kahn, A. (2001). Frontal lobe changes in alcoholism: A review of the literature. *Alcohol and Alcoholism, 36*(5), 357–368.

[22] Oscar-Berman, M., & Hutner, N. (1993). Frontal lobe changes after chronic alcohol ingestion. In W. A. Hunt, & S. J. Nixon (Eds.), *Alcohol-induced brain damage* (pp. 121–156). Rockville, MD: NIAA. vol. Monograph No. 22.

[23] Oscar-Berman, M., & Marinkovic, K. (2003). Alcoholism and the brain: An overview. *Alcohol Research and Health, 27*(2), 125–133.

[24] Sullivan, E. V. (2003). Compromised pontocerebellar and cerebellothalamocorticalsystems: Speculations on their contributions to cognitiveand motor impairment in nonamnesic alcoholism. *Alcoholism: Clinical and Experimental Research, 27*(9), 1409–1419.

[25] Bates, M. E., & Convit, A. (1999). Neuropsychology and neuroimaging of alcohol and illicit drug abuse. In A. Calev (Ed.), *Assessment of neuropsychological functions in psychiatric disorders* (pp. 373–445). Washington: American Psychiatric Press.

[26] Noel, X., Linden, V. M., & Schnidt, N. (2001). Supervisory attentional system in non amnestic alcoholic men. *Archives of General Psychiatry, 58*(12), 1152–1180.

[27] Zinn, S., Stein, R., & Swartzwelder, H. S. (2004). Executive functioning early in abstinence from alcohol. *Alcoholism, Clinical and Experimental Research, 28*(9), 1338–1346.

[28] Hughes, J. R., & John, E. R. (1999). Conventional and quantitative electroencephalography in psychiatry. *The Journal of Neuropsychiatry and Clinical Neurosciences, 11*, 190–208.

[29] Hammond, D. C. (2001). Treatment of chronic fatigue with neurofeedback and self hypnosis. *NeuroRehabilitation, 16*, 295–300.

[30] Peniston, E. G., & Kulkosky, P. J. (1989). Alpha–theta brainwave training and beta-endorphin levels in alcoholics. *Alcoholism, Clinical and Experimental Research, 13*(2), 271–279.

[31] Saxby, E., & Peniston, E. G. (1995). Alpha–theta brainwave neurofeedback training: An effective treatment for male and female alcoholics with depressive symptoms. *Journal of Clinical Psychology, 51*(5), 685–693.

[32] Klimesch, W. (1999). EEG alpha and theta oscillations reflect cognitive and memory performance: A review and analysis. *Brain Research Reviews, 29*(2–3), 169–195.

[33] Hanslmayr, S., Sauseng, P., Doppelmayr, M., Schabus, M., & Klimesch, W. (2005). Increasing individual upper alpha power by neurofeedback improves cognitive performance in human subjects. *Applied Psychophysiology and Biofeedback, 30*(1), 1–10.

[34] Hebert, R., Lehmann, D., Tan, G., Travis, F., & Arenander, A. (2005). Enhanced EEG alpha time- domain phase synchrony during transcendental meditation: Implications for cortical integration theory. *Signal Processing Archive*, *85*(11), 2213–2232.

[35] Passini, F. T., Watson, C. G., & Herder, J. (1978). Alpha biofeedback therapy in alcoholics: An 18 month follow up. *Journal of Clinical Psychology*, *34*(3), 765–769.

[36] Scott, W. C., Kaiser, D., Othmer, S., & Sideroff, S. I. (2005). Effect of an EEG biofeedback training protocol on a mixed substance abusing population. *The American Journal of Drug and Alcohol Abuse*, *31*, 455–469.

[37] Thomas, S., Rajeswaran, J., & Murthy, P. (2009). *Neurofeedback training in alcohol dependent individuals*. Ph.D.Thesis. Bangalore: National Institute of Mental Health And Neurosciences (Deemed University)

[38] Hyder, A. A., Wunderlich, C. A., Puvanchandra, P., Gururaj, G., & Kobusingya, O. C. (2007). The impact of traumatic brain injuries: A global perspective. *NeuroRehabilitation*, *22*(5), 341–353.

[39] Reilly, P. (2007). The impact of neurotrauma on society: An international perspective. *Progress in Brain Research*, *161*, 3–9.

[40] Thorell, W., & Aarabi, B. (2001). History of neurosurgical techniques in head injury. *Neurosurgery Clinics of North America*, *12*, 11–22.

[41] Gururaj, G. (2002). Epidemiology of traumatic brain injuries: An Indian scenario. *Neuorological Research*, *24*, 24–28.

[42] Whitfield, P. C., Thomas, E. O., Summers, F., Whyte, M., & Hutchinson, P. J. (2009). *Head injury: A multidisciplinary approach*. Cambridge University Press.

[43] Lishman, A. (1998). *Organic psychiatry: The psychological consequences of cerebral disorder*. London: Blackwell.

[44] Heegaard, W., & Biros, M. (2006). Head injury. In J. Marx, R. Hockberger, & R. Walls (Eds.), *Rosen's emergency medicine* (pp. 349–382) (6 eds.). Philadelphia: Mosby/Elsevier.

[45] Granacher, R. P., Jr. (2008). Commentary: Applications of functional neuroimaging to civil litigation of mild traumatic brain injury. *Journal of American Academic Psychiatry Law*, *36*, 323–328.

[46] Stuss, D. T., Stethem, L. L., Hugenholtz, H., Picton, T., Pivik, J., & Richard, M. T. (1989). Reaction time after head injury: Fatigue, divided and focused attention, and consistency of performance. *Journal of Neurology Neurosurgery and Psychiatry*, *52*, 742–748.

[47] Leclercq, M., Couillet, J., Azouvi, P., Marlier, N., Martin, Y., Strypstein, E., et al. (2000). Dual task performance after severe diffuse traumatic brain injury or vascular prefrontal damage. *Journal of Clinical and Experimental Neuropsychology*, *22*, 339–350.

[48] Whyte, J., Schuster, K., Polansky, M., Adams, J., & Coslett, H. B. (2000). Frequency and duration of inattentive behaviour after traumatic brain injury: Effects of distraction, task, and practice. *Journal of the International Neuropsychological Society*, *6*, 1–11.

[49] McAvinue, L., O'Keeffe, F., McMackin, D., & Robertson, I. H. (2005). Impaired sustained attention and error awareness in traumatic brain injury: Implications for insight. *Neuropsychological Rehabilitation*, *15*, 569–587.

[50] Madigan, N. K., DeLuca, J., Diamond, B. J., Tramontano, G., & Averill, A. (2000). Speed of information processing in traumatic brain injury: Modality-specific factors. *Journal of Head Trauma Rehabililation*, *15*, 943–956.

[51] Rassovsky, Y., Satz, P., Alfano, M. S., Light, R. K., Zaucha, K., Mcarthur, D. L., et al. (2006). Functional outcome in TBI II: Verbal memory and information processing speed

mediators come in TBI II. *Journal of Clinical and Experimental Neuropsychology, 28,* 581–591.

[52] Serino, A., Ciaramelli, E., Di Santantonio, A., Malagu, S., Servadei, F., & Ladavas, E. (2006). Central executive system impairment in traumatic brain injury. *Brain Injury, 20,* 23–32.

[53] Dikmen, S. S., Machamer, J. E., Powell, J. M., & Temkin, N. R. (2003). Outcome 3 to 5 years after moderate to severe traumatic brain injury. *Archives of Physical Medicine and Rehabilitation, 84,* 1449–1457.

[54] Kersel, D. A., Marsh, N. V., Mars, V., Havill, J. H., & Sleigh, J. W. (2001). Neuropsychological functioning during the year following severe traumatic brain injury. *Brain Injury, 15,* 283–296.

[55] Temkin, N. R., Machamer, J. E., & Dikmen, S. S. (2003). Correlates of functional status 3–5 years after traumatic brain injury with CT abnormalities. *Journal of Neurotrauma, 20,* 229–241.

[56] Reddy, R. P., Rajan, J., Bagavathula, I., & Kandavel, T. (2009). Neurofeedback training to enhance learning and memory in patient with traumatic brain injury: A single case study. *International Journal of Psychosocial Rehabilitation, 14,* 21–28.

[57] Hanks, R. A., Rapport, L. J., Millis, S. R., & Deshpande, S. A. (1999). Measures of executive functioning as predictors of functional ability and social integration in a rehabilitation sample. *Archives of Physical and Medical Rehabilitation, 80,* 1030–1037.

[58] Jamuna, N. (2007). A comprehensive approach to neuropsychological rehabilitation. In K. Rao (Ed.), *Mindscapes, global perspectives on psychology in mental health* (pp. 307–314). Bangalore: NIMHANS.

[59] Ayers, M. E. (1987). Electroencephalographic neurofeedback and closed head injury of 250 individuals. In *National head injury syllabus*. Washington, DC: National Head Injury Foundation. (pp. 380–392).

[60] Thatcher, R. W., Walker, R. A., Gerson, I., & Geisler, F. H. (1989). EEG discriminant analyses of mild head trauma. *Electroencephalography Clinical Neurophysiology, 73,* 94–106.

[61] Peniston, E. G., Marrinan, D. A., Deming, W. A., & Kulkosky, P. J. (1993). EEG alpha-theta synchronization in Vietnam theater veterans with combat-related post-traumatic stress disorder and alcohol abuse. *Advances in Medical Psychotherapy, 6,* 37–50.

[62] Hoffman, D. A., Stockdale, S., Hicks, L. L., & Schwaninger, J. E. (1995). Diagnosis and treatment of head injury. *Journal of Neurotherapy, 1,* 14–21.

[63] Rozelle, G. R., & Budzynski, T. H. (1995). Neurotherapy for stroke rehabilitation: A single case study. *Biofeedback Self Regulation, 20,* 211–228.

[64] Hoffman, D. A., Stockdale, S., Hicks, L. L., & Schwaninger, J. E. (1995). Diagnosis and treatment of head injury. *Journal of Neurotherapy, 1,* 14–21.

[65] Ham, L. P., & Packard, R. C. (1996). A retrospective, follow up study of biofeedback assisted relaxation therapy in patients with post traumatic head ache. *Biofeedback Self Regulation, 21*(2), 93–104.

[66] Thornton, K. (2000). Improvement/rehabilitation of memory functioning with neurotherapy/QEEG biofeedback. *Journal of Head Trauma Rehabilitation, 15,* 1285–1296.

[67] Keller, K. (2001). Neurofeedback therapy of attention deficits in patients with traumatic brain injury. *Journal of Neurotherapy, 5*(1/2).

[68] Zelek, V. (2008). QEEG brainwave amplitude and coherence values as predictors of cognitive improvement to neurofeedback after moderate-to-severe acquired brain injury. In North American brain injury society's sixth annual conference on brain injury. New

Orleans, LA: Lippincott Williams & Wilkins, Inc, (Abstract: *Journal of Head Trauma Rehabilitation*, 23, 343).

[69] Oldfield, R. C. (1971). The assessment and analysis of handedness: The Edinburgh inventory. *Neuopsychologia*, *9*, 97–113.

[70] Rao, S. L., Subbakrishna, D. K., & Gopukumar, K. (2004). *NIMHANS neuropsychology battery—2004*. Bangalore: NIMHANS Publication.

[71] King, N. S., Crawford, S., Wenden, F. J., Moss, N. E., & Wade, D. T. (1995). The rivermead post concussion symptoms questionnaire: A measure of symptoms commonly experienced after head injury and its reliability. *Journal of Neurology*, *1242*, 587–592.

[72] Crawford, S., Wenden, F. J., & Wade, D. T. (1996). The rivermead head injury follow up questionnaire: A study of a new rating scale and other measures to evaluate outcome after head injury. *Journal of Neurology, Neurosurgery, and Psychiatry*, *60*, 510–514.

[73] WHO Group, (1994). Development of the WHOQOL rational and current status. *International Journal of Mental Health*, *2*, 24–56.

[74] Duffy, F. H. (2000). The State of EEG Biofeedback therapy (EEG prerant conditioning) in 2000: An editors opinion. *Clinical Electroencephalography*, *31*(1), v–viii. editorial.

[75] Manchesler, C. F., Allen, T., & Tachiki, K. H. (1998). Treatment of dissociative identity disorder with neurotherapy and group self exploration. *Neurotherapy*, *2*(4), 40–52.

[76] Banerjee, D. (2006). Epidemiology of stroke in India. *Neurology Asia*, *11*, 1–4.

[77] Gourie-Devi, M., Gururaj, G., Satishchandra, P., & Subbakrishna, D. K. (2004). Prevalence of neurological disorders in Bangalore, India. *A Community-based study with a comparison between urban and rural areas. Neuroepidemiology*, *23*, 261–268.

[78] Phillips, N., Mate-Kole, C., & Kirby, R. (1993). Neuropsychological function in peripheral vascular disease amputee patients. *Archives of Physical Medicine and Rehabilitation*, *74*, 1309–1314.

[79] Kauhanen, M., Korpelainen, J. T., Hiltunen, P., Brusin, E., Mononen, H., Maatta, R., et al. (1999). Poststroke depression correlates with cognitive impairment and neurological deficits. *Stroke*, *30*(9), 1875–1880.

[80] Strauss, E., Sherman, E. M. S., & Spreen, O. (2006). *A Compendium of neuropsychological tests: Administration, norms, and Commentary*. Oxford: Oxford University Press.

[81] Lezak, M. D. (2004). *Neuropsychological Assessment*. Oxford: Oxford University Press.

# 5 Applications of Cognitive Behavioral Principles in Neuropsychological Rehabilitation

*P.M. Sudhir*

Department of Clinical Psychology, National Institute of Mental Health and Neurosciences (NIMHANS), Bangalore, Karnataka, India

## Introduction

Traumatic brain injuries (TBIs) are a leading cause of death and disability the world over, the majority affecting the population in early adulthood. Nearly 15% of survivors continue to experience symptoms beyond 3 years [1]. The socioemotional and behavioral disturbances following TBI are a major cause of concern for the patient and the family. Behavior disorders are said to be the most enduring and socially disabling of the problems seen typically after brain injury [2]. Managing maladaptive behavior due to disorders of motivation or personality change is one of the most important goals of neuropsychological rehabilitation. The disturbances that follow TBI are a function of an interaction of several factors, including premorbid cognitive and social skills, the nature of the brain injury and its consequences, and the social environment following injury. Individuals who have suffered TBI have higher rates of psychiatric problems, difficulties in handling emotions and day-to-day emotional and social demands. As a result, their social world shrinks, contributing further to social withdrawal. Neuropsychological or cognitive rehabilitation is described as a set of therapeutic procedures that are based on brain-behavior relationships. It consists of reestablishing or reinforcing patterns of behavior that were previously established, establishing cognitive activity through cognitive mechanisms, using external mechanisms and establishing new activities, and helping the individual adapt to the cognitive disability by improving overall functioning [3].

The four main domains of rehabilitation recognized are restitution, substitution, activation, and integration, each of which requires different therapeutic strategies of varying complexity. The integration of functions is one of the ultimate aims of neuropsychological rehabilitation, and this requires the use of specific training programs to ensure interaction between various modules that have already been carried out.

In a conference of the Association for the Advancement of Behavior Therapy, held in Chicago in 1978, Horton [4] coined the term "behavioral neuropsychology."

Neuropsychological Rehabilitation-Principles and Applications.
DOI: http://dx.doi.org/10.1016/B978-0-12-416046-0.00005-5

Behavioral neuropsychology was defined as "… application of behavior therapy techniques to problems of organically impaired individuals while using a neuropsychological assessment and intervention perspective." This definition is an important recognition of integration of behavioral principles and methods with the neuropsychological perspective of organic impairment. While the neuropsychological perspective will help in understanding the impairments, the behavioral assessment would additionally distinguish the various excess and deficit behaviors that can be targeted in therapy. Maladaptive behavior is one aspect or facet of a complex neurobehavioral picture.

Learning is important at every step of the neuropsychological rehabilitation program. Brain injury interferes with learning in several ways: by hampering information processing, by not allowing for integration of information; and by disrupting the cognitive functions necessary for integration to occur, such as attention, perception, and judgment [5,6]. In order to develop effective programs for rehabilitation, it is necessary to understand the estimate of learning difficulties and then devise a set of strategies to help the person overcome them. The program should additionally identify alternate skills and ways of learning, and should plan generalization of these skills to community living [7].

Various similarities have been noted between the neuropsychological assessment following brain injury and behavioral neuropsychology. The first common interest is the focus on the functional and ecological validity of the evaluation. This is done in order to facilitate transfer of gains in relevant behaviors to the patient's natural environment, by designing a program for functional rehabilitation of daily life. The main aim of evaluation is treatment, and hence the two (neuropsychological assessment and behavioral neuropsychology) are complementary to each other [8,9]. Knowledge of the functional demands of the patient, the resources that will be available, and the limitations is very important to build a program. As a result of this evaluation, an individual formulation and treatment plan is drawn up, consisting of maintaining antecedents or stimulus cues and consequences. Several authors have described the use of functional analysis as well as the formulation of treatment plans based on learning principles [10–13].

The combination of the neuropsychological perspective with behavioral techniques offers an advantage to the therapist managing patients with behavioral, emotional, and social functioning problems [14]. Behavior modification, or the application of operant procedures to the modification of behaviors, is an effective method to eliminate, alter, or modify undesirable behaviors while increasing the probability of adaptive behaviors.

Behavior therapy is an applied discipline that has made significant contributions to the field of rehabilitation; its primary focus is on measurable behavior [15]. Acquisition and maintenance of problem behaviors are explained using learning theory. In addition to acquisition and maintenance, the behavioral paradigm also explains mechanisms by which the therapist can strengthen old patterns and eliminate inappropriate behaviors by altering antecedents and consequences.

Behavior disorders often represent a significant barrier to effective rehabilitation of cognitive dysfunction. They can hamper other interventions due to the patient being aggressive, apathetic, and amotivated. Therefore, it is important to address these issues and ensure that the individual benefits from the rehabilitation program. It goes beyond improving cognitive functions into becoming more adaptive and functional in daily life. Therapeutic interventions that are based on neuropsychological interventions are more holistic and integrated when they include strategies to deal with maladaptive behaviors. The challenge for the therapist is to rehabilitate in the least restrictive way possible. According to Horton and Howe [16], the "blend of neuropsychology and behavior therapy can produce an effective treatment program for a certain percentage of brain injured individuals." Ben-Yishay and Gold [17] describe holistic neuropsychological interventions as those "interventions that are directed at the remediation of cognitive deficits, emotional mastery, interpersonal communication and social competencies and acceptance of the consequences of the brain injury within the context of a therapeutic community. The aims of psychotherapeutic interventions along with neuropsychological interventions are manifold. They help patient accept certain changes that are irreversible, such as the loss of a function, or develop an alternate lifestyle, build coping strategies that would enhance mastery and reduce distress as well as reduce distressing behaviors and increase activation through specific behavioral and motivational procedures."

## Components of Applied Behavior Analysis

Effective applied behavior analysis (ABA) is a powerful tool for teaching people appropriate ways of interacting with their environment. ABA and the resulting behavior modification program are based on the operant-conditioning principle that asserts that human behavior is continuously modified by the environment depending on the consequences of one's behavior. The terms behavior modification and operant procedures are often used interchangeably in the literature. They consist of structured procedures aimed at either reducing behaviors that are disruptive or maladaptive or at increasing actions that empower a person. Behavioral approaches have specifically targeted practical and specific overt behaviors.

One of the important features of a behavioral program is the functional analysis and identification of maintaining antecedents for inappropriate behaviors. The functional analysis forms the first and most important step in the formulation of a behavioral program. A behavioral evaluation, the detailed Antecedent Behavior Consequence (ABC) analysis of behavioral deficits and excesses, is necessary for the choice and implementation of a suitable therapeutic plan.

The breaking up of larger behaviors into smaller units based on principles such as chaining and setting subgoals is important in reducing task difficulty and sequentially arranging cues for target behaviors. From a behavioral analysis perspective, disorders can be categorized as (1) excesses (in which something is in addition to the normal repertoire of behavior, e.g., aggression, self-stimulation, and verbally abusive behavior); (2) deficits (lack of specific social skills, inability to take care of self, incontinence, and inability to play the role expected); (3) inappropriate stimulus control (behavior occurs at the wrong place or time); and (4) disorders such as depression or paranoia. Deficits refer to an absence or reduced intensity or frequency of required behaviors/skills. These span various areas such as social skills, self-help skills, self-regulatory behaviors, and so on. Identifying deficits would help in planning programs that would facilitate or increase these behaviors.

Individuals with head injuries present with a heterogeneous nature of deficits, and these include impairments in functions such as social skill deficits, motoric impairments, and excesses including aggressive or inappropriate behaviors. Despite this heterogeneity, researchers and clinicians note that behavioral techniques are effective for patients with brain injuries. The various problems for which behavior therapy has been found to be effective include aggression; socially inappropriate behaviors; amotivation; motor impairment, including spasticity, muscle strength, and movement; and speech impairments such as dysarthria, as well as to enhance activities of daily living (ADL). In addition, the principles of behavior therapy such as shaping, prompting massed practice, and so on are also applied to the implementation of traditional neuropsychological rehabilitation programs [18]. Studies of neuropsychological rehabilitation that included behavioral and social interventions have reported greater effect sizes than those without such techniques [19,20].

Behavioral assessment allows the clinician to discriminate between behaviors maintained by environmental contingencies and those that occur due to brain injury or that are a result of skill deficit [21]. A naturalistic observation is best suited to obtain an accurate sample of behaviors. Observations over several occasions and situations in addition to the reports of significant others provide the clinician the necessary information to formulate a treatment program. Observation of the patient in natural settings also allows the therapist to identify antecedents that may not be evident in the clinical setting.

## Models for Assessment

Glasgow et al. [22] developed a model for the evaluation of deficits in memory in patients with brain damage. The evaluation under this model comprises four parts, including a general evaluation of neuropsychological functioning and a comparison with other patients with similar characteristics. It includes a specific behavioral evaluation of the problem and the patient. The objective of this assessment is to understand the parameters of the patient's behavior, using functional analysis of behavior, and an assessment of the generalization of treatment effects to ADL. The last two sections of the evaluation are related to the intervention program.

Godoy [23] proposed a seven-phase model of behavioral neuropsychology very similar to the ABC analysis. This model includes an evaluation of the general state of the patient, the present behavioral alterations (cognitive–affective–emotional deficits or excesses, motor problems, and physiological or psychosocial dysfunctions in their most relevant parameters such as frequency, duration, and intensity), and the abilities or resources that are still present. The next two phases involve the identification of the internal as well as external, and antecedent and consequent, variables that aggravate or alleviate the target problems; the consequences of the disease on a personal, familiar, social, and vocational level are evaluated. In the fourth and fifth phases, information and perceptions about the problems, causes, symptoms, and treatment are enquired into, along with the motivation of the patient to initiate treatment and further continue with the intervention. The family's willingness to cooperate in the rehabilitation process is evaluated. Finally, the model includes periodic assessments of the program and adherence by the patient. Behavioral neuropsychology is thus a distinct area from classical neuropsychological evaluation; from the start, it adapts functional criteria of evaluation and the entire evaluation is oriented toward planning treatment.

The major advantages of behavioral and cognitive behavioral programs lie in their highly structured format, and in fact, they are amenable to specialized adaptation to memory, attention, and problem-solving impairments [24]. Reintegration into the community requires complex social and behavioral skills that may be affected in individuals with TBI. Behavioral, cognitive, and social interventions provide these skills to the individual.

Goal setting is another important issue in the behavioral assessment of patients with brain injuries. The assessment of behaviors as well as the goals to be achieved in rehabilitation must take into account the patient's natural environment. This ensures that goals set are reasonable and that the patient will be able to utilize the skills acquired in his/her own environment and will be reinforced for it [25].

# Application of Reinforcement Principles in Neuropsychological Rehabilitation

Operant principles are perhaps the most widely used among the behavior therapy strategies [18]. Operant procedures are based on the manipulation of consequences, either by providing rewards contingent on appropriate behavior (positive programming) or the withdrawal of rewards or reinforcing environments contingent on inappropriate behaviors (response cost or time out). Reinforcement refers to any stimulus or event whose presence increases the probability of occurrence of a behavior. Reinforcements have been widely used to modify undesirable behaviors such as aggression. Despite the fact that patients with TBI may have cognitive deficits, learning is not hampered when concrete reinforcements are used.

The withdrawal of rewards leads to a decrease in the probability of the occurrence of an undesired behavior. Some commonly used techniques include response cost or withdrawal of rewards or tokens earned, and time out, which involves the removal of the person from a pleasant/neutral environment to a nonreinforcing environment. Response cost is a cognitive behavioral technique based on the operant principle of contingent punishment, or negative punishment, and has been used to enhance behavioral control. Alderman and Burgess [26] report the use of response cost along with cognitive overlearning in a patient with herpes encephalitis, who demonstrated repetitive speech and other problems of poor social skills, as well as incontinence.

Schedules of reinforcement determine the manner in which reinforcements will be delivered. They allow greater discrimination of cues, such as the use of differential reinforcement. These involve the manipulation of antecedent cues and thereby reduction or elimination of behaviors that occur exclusively in response to cues. The success of operant procedures is based on the careful and detailed analysis of the behaviors as well as the settings in which they occur and factors that maintain them. The criterion for success with reference to target behaviors must also be specified (such as frequency of an appropriate behavior and magnitude).

Serno [18] provides a detailed discussion of the main behavior modifications and their applications, as well as limitations to neuropsychological rehabilitation. Some of the main techniques highlighted in this review are the use of positive reinforcement, prompts, cues, and fading in the management of aphasia, and the use of response hierarchies, shaping, and differential reinforcement in the management of stereotyped verbal responses. Programmed therapy is another contribution of the operant school of learning to rehabilitation programs. In a programmed progression, response hierarchies are created, and cues and prompts to be delivered are also determined.

Accelerative techniques are those techniques that increase the frequency or intensity of target behaviors, whereas decelerative behaviors are those that help decrease the frequency or intensity of target behaviors. Accelerative behavioral techniques include positive programming, shaping, and chaining; decelerative techniques include differential reinforcement of incompatible behavior, other behaviors (DRO), and low-rate behaviors, overcorrection, stimulus change, stimulus satiation or massed practice, time out, and response cost. Complex strategies include contingency contracting, stimulus control, and token economy.

The most researched area in the behavioral management of TBI is the management of aggression and other behavioral disturbances that occur as a consequence of TBI, such as self-injurious behaviors. Aggressive behavior is one of the most disturbing consequences and is a serious hindrance to the progress of rehabilitation as it hampers the use of other rehabilitation strategies and interferes with the social functioning of the patient. Frequently used behavioral strategies in the management of aggression and behavioral disturbances include the use of positive reinforcement and modeling [27], differential reinforcement and token economy [28–30], overcorrection and restitution [31,32], and time out and response cost [26]. Some studies have also used a combination of strategies such as self-monitoring of anxiety, cognitive restructuring, and instrumental mastery skills [33]. It must be noted that the most effective behavior therapy programs are a combination of both decelerative and accelerative techniques, rather than the isolated use of strategies. Punishment and other aversive techniques are used based on the principle of the least coercive methods and are rarely used in the absence of positive programming strategies. Thus, while one target behavior is on a deceleration program, such as response cost or time out, a desirable target behavior identified in the ABC analysis is placed on a positive reinforcement schedule. This ensures that while maladaptive behaviors are eliminated or decreased, the patient has an opportunity to develop an adaptive repertoire as well.

Aggression has also been managed by changing antecedents of aggression, decreasing stimulation, increasing predictability by scheduling, signaling an impending event, and approaching a patient from a side that is not affected by visual neglect. Management of inappropriate behaviors, including nonverbal activities such as throat clearing, spitting, hoarding, and verbal behaviors such as screaming, shouting, and complaining, have been effectively managed with straightforward reinforcement methods such as DRO and other methods such as the contingent withdrawal of rewards through time out and response cost.

Alderman and Burgess [26] report the use of response cost along with cognitive overlearning in a patient with herpes encephalitis who demonstrated repetitive speech. Burgess and Alderman [33] describe the use of response cost and training in self-monitoring in patients with prefrontal lobe lesions who had problems such as verbal abuse, poor social skills, and urinary incontinence.

One of the major difficulties with the use of operant procedures in the management of behavioral disturbances resulting from TBI is the maintenance of gains in the natural environment. Often the cues and contingencies present in the patient's natural environment do not support changes. One way in which these difficulties can be overcome is through the involvement of significant others in treatment programs. In cultures where the patient continues to stay in the home with families and is not under hospital care alone, this is a promising method.

Similarly, token economy systems have been used to modify several behaviors within a complex program [34]. Alderman and Knight [35] report the use of differential reinforcement in dealing with physically aggressive behavior in a patient following TBI. In a single case study with multiple baseline assessment, Hegel and Ferguson [36] report using differential reinforcement in a young man with TBI and aggressive behaviors as sequelae. In differential reinforcement, the undesirable behavior is placed on an extinction schedule, while the desired behavior is positively reinforced.

Becker and Vakil [37] describe the steps in a behavioral program adopted to treat two types of frontal lobe syndromes called disinhibition and adynamia. The steps outlined include establishing a therapeutic alliance, diagnostic evaluation, identification of target problems, implementation of the behavioral strategies including contingency contracting, reinforcement, relaxation training, social skills, and rehearsal and role plays. The final steps in this program include the generalization of skills to naturalistic settings. According to the authors, these patients with frontal lobe injury lacked sensitivity to feedback; the behavioral strategy of manipulating the environment provides this feedback. The exaggerated reinforcements that are provided help in building adaptive mechanisms.

# Social Skills Training

Social skills intervention is based on the assumption that problems in social interaction are a result of inadequately developed knowledge of relevant social rules. As a result, social skills programs have focused on training individuals in socially relevant behaviors such as communication skills, assertiveness, and negotiation skills. Individuals with TBI may, however, lack some of the basic prerequisites for effective social skills training to occur, such as motivation, ability to transfer knowledge to natural settings, and self-regulation [19]. In the context of TBI, social skills training includes skills to improve conversational ability, assertion, amount of interaction, and personal appearance. Social skills training has been carried out using prompts, fading, reinforcement contingencies, modeling, shaping, time out for inappropriate talk, feedback, self-management, problem solving, role plays, and social problem solving. Other procedures used are discrimination training, rehearsal, and practice [19].

Structured social skills training in the form of communication skills exercises has been applied to improve the social behavior of patients. Group skills training for patients with left hemisphere stroke with aphasia was reported in one study. In this study, one group received group communication skills while the other group was placed in the deferred treatment group. The results of their study supported the use of group communication skills that involved specific tasks and generalization in patients with aphasia. The use of role plays and problem solving along with functional communication skills training has also been described to be helpful in rehabilitation of speech impairments [19].

## Other Behavior Therapy Procedures in TBI

Relaxation training is an effective technique in reducing muscle tension. Muscle tension in some situations is learned and associated with actual physical effort or psychological stress. Relaxation can be achieved through several strategies such as deep muscle relaxation, diaphragmatic breathing, or biofeedback training. One study reported the effectiveness of relaxation training in increasing syntax stimulation. Aeschleman and Imes [38] report a case series in which they used stress inoculation including relaxation training, coping skills, and self-instruction in individuals with TBI.

Constraint-induced therapy (CIT) is another recent example of the application of learning theory and behavior therapy to cognitive rehabilitation. It has been used in both movement therapy and speech therapy. CIT is a set of techniques based on studies carried out on primates. It includes conditioned response training, shaping, and other behavioral strategies that are effective in overcoming learned nonuse [39]. Constraint-induced speech therapy is described as a massed practice of verbal responses and is designed to restrict or constrain the patient to systematic practice [40].

Ylvisaker et al. [19] reviewed the various behavioral and social interventions for individuals with TBI. They highlight two major but overlapping interventions that have emerged since the introduction of applied behavior analysis (ABA). Apart from the traditional ABA, positive behavior support (PBS) is also recognized as an emerging and promising approach to the management of TBI. In their comparison between the two approaches, they note that while ABA focuses on modification of behaviors by the manipulation of identified antecedents and consequences within a controlled and possibly experimental situation, the PBS approach is more focused on lifestyle changes and accepts that the most effective way to manage behavior is by organizing immediate and remote antecedent support so that individuals are likely to behave successfully and, with practice, acquire repertoires of behavior that enable them to succeed in their social contexts. PBS also focuses on errorless learning, a concept that is discussed in neuropsychological rehabilitation as well. As PBS is still an emerging approach, there is still a lot more research to be carried out to establish its efficacy. The authors list various tasks including support communication, task planning, daily routines, and so on. Studies combine PBS with tradition ABA to implement multicomponent interventions. The major difficulty with multicomponent interventions is that it is difficult to determine the individual impact of various interventions [19,20].

## Biofeedback and Neuropsychological Rehabilitation

Biofeedback is a set of therapeutic procedures based on operant learning. It involves the modification of involuntary, physiological, and motor responses with the help of feedback. The application of biofeedback involves the use of specific learning principles such as discrimination training, shaping, and reinforcement through knowledge of results. It is a procedure that is based on the principle of self-regulation. The use of electromyography (EMG) biofeedback in rehabilitation programs aimed at reducing physical disability caused by TBI or other neurological conditions has been well researched. EMG biofeedback has been used extensively in the management of spasticity, paresis, and apraxias [41,42].

A relatively new and promising approach in cognitive rehabilitation, particularly for TBI, is electroencephalogram (EEG) biofeedback. The therapeutic application of EEG biofeedback is often referred to as neurofeedback or neurotherapy. EEG biofeedback is an operant-conditioning procedure that aims to modify and normalize dysregulated EEG patterns [43–46]. There is a small but growing body of evidence that indicates that EEG biofeedback interventions have proved to be useful in remediating cognitive difficulties in patients with TBI for various problems such as anger, headaches, memory, cognitive flexibility, mood, attention, and cognitive performance deficits, and for normalization of EEG patterns [47–52]. Controlled studies such as that by Thornton [53] indicate that the effects of EEG biofeedback may also be seen in terms of reduced use of medication. Methodological limitations, including a lack of functional outcomes, follow-up, and simultaneous use of other cognitive rehabilitation methods have limited the generalizability of these findings.

## Applications of Behavioral and Cognitive Behavioral Programs in Self- and Emotion Regulation

The role of cognitive and behavioral interventions in the rehabilitation of higher cognitive processes such as self- and emotion-regulation skills and other executive functions has been studied by many researchers in recent years. Self-regulation is at the core of executive functions. Self-regulatory behavior is mediated by the frontal lobe. It is a set of dynamic relationships between metacognitive beliefs and knowledge, ongoing self-monitoring and self-assessment during activities, and self-control (strategy decisions) [54–56]. Metacognition is also a topic of research interest with respect to emotional disorders and their treatments [57]. The role of these cognitive processes in more complex behavior is well established. Among the higher mental functions, reasoning and problem solving are considered to be the most complex. Both these functions require prerequisites such as adequate motivation, attention, use of feedback for self-monitoring of performance, and the capacity to evaluate one's own performance [58]. Impairments in these functions can cause several difficulties to the individual in carrying out day-to-day tasks. Milder levels of impairment may not be obvious, but gross impairments can cause disruption in even basic ADL such as keeping appointments and managing financial matters such as bills and banking [59]. There is a considerable degree of overlap between the cognitive behavioral and neuropsychological conceptualizations of problem-solving skills as both involve a step-by-step approach using various other cognitive tasks such as generating alternatives, decision making, and so on. While the cognitive behavioral perspective assumes a macrolevel understanding of problem solving, the neuropsychologist takes on a more microlevel view.

Baddeley and Wilson [60] describe the *dysexecution syndrome* as the functional deficits of patients with prefrontal lobe lesions. It includes the impairment in memory, inertia of thinking, disorders of planning and thinking, motivation, and mental tension during the execution of a task [61]. Motivational disturbances are a cause of major concern following brain injury. They affect the perception and solution of problems [62]. Thus, cognitive rehabilitation programs that are designed to enhance motivation are very important.

Behavior modification techniques have been found to be an effective way to improve motivation in patients with brain injuries. The major behavioral techniques that have been found to be effective include token economy systems, positive reinforcement, time out for inappropriate behaviors, and differential reinforcements to reduce maladaptive behaviors and increase adaptive ones.

Problem solving has been defined as a set of goal-directed cognitive activities that arises in situations for which there is no immediately apparent or available response [63,64]. In such situations, the individual must use cognitive skills to go beyond the information given to find a solution to the problem at hand [65]. The application of problem solving in emotional disorders is well established. However, in a manner that has significance for cognitive or neuropsychological rehabilitation, this view of problem-solving skills has been revised to accommodate the neuropsychological perspective [66,67]. The modified definition of problem-solving skills stresses those aspects of the process that "disrupt and thereby interfere with problem solving performance" [68]. Cognitive behavior therapy (CBT) addresses problem solving at a macro level and in this way differs from the approach taken by neuropsychological rehabilitation. It incorporates motivational, attitudinal, and affective aspects of real-life problem resolution.

Each step in problem solving involves a series of self-regulatory as well as emotion-regulation skills. Effective social problem solving plays an important role in the processing of information about self, others, and the environment [69]. In individuals already vulnerable to emotional dysregulation, the negative emotions associated with problems are likely to be more intense. Emotional dysregulation has also been identified as a predictor of community integration [70]. Individuals with deficits in executive functions may also have slower speeds of processing and many may already be experiencing information overload [71]. Using this rationale, Rath et al. [67] conducted a study in which 60 individuals with head injury were trained in problem-solving and emotion-regulation strategies. The innovative treatment consisted of twelve 2-h sessions focused on reducing the factors that hampered effective problem solving such as cognitive distortions and misattributions, as well as on improving self-efficacy. The techniques were based on cognitive behavioral principles and included verbal challenging and correction of negative self-talk. The results of the study indicated significant improvements in the group receiving the innovative treatment in problem solving, self-appraisal, executive functions, self-appraised clear thinking, and emotion regulation and role-playing scenarios.

In an earlier study, Cicerone and Giacino [71] demonstrated the effects of making predictions and getting feedback, that is, effects of self-instruction with feedback and self-monitoring therapy. They found that with self-monitoring therapy, five of six participants had fewer errors and less off-task behavior after therapy. During self-monitoring therapy, performance improved with feedback, but decreased again when feedback was withdrawn, indicating the effect of feedback on performance. Similarly, Suzman et al. [72] used several components of cognitive behavioral therapy to improve problem-solving skills in children with TBI. This included self-instruction and regulation, metacognitive strategies, attribution training, and feedback as reinforcement. Children produced fewer errors while solving problems during a computerized game, although the researchers did not distinguish between therapy components or phases. Kennedy et al. [56] reviewed intervention studies for self-regulation. They reviewed 15 studies that focused on some aspect of problem solving, planning, organization, and multitasking, including social [56,68] or behavioral problem solving, time management, goal management, generating solutions, and decision making [73–77]; planning using self-regulation during complex problem activities [78,79]; verbal reasoning [79–81]; continuing complex activities with cues [82]; using organization strategies during functional activities [83]; and dual-task training [84]. Instructional training and problem solving have thus shown promise in improving planning, organization, and other self-regulation skills [78,83]. However, these studies have significant methodological limitations, many of them being single case designs.

Fasotti [85], in a review of executive function retraining, highlights the importance of self-instruction training and cueing in patients with self-regulation skills deficits. The use of goal management training (GMT) based on the theory of neglect [84] has been reported [75]. GMT is a step-by-step approach involving setting goals and subgoals through a series of problem-solving questions and self-instruction, similar to the goal setting used in behavioral programs.

In their review, Cicerone et al. [84] present studies using cueing and external contingencies as well as response cost for improving behavioral and emotional regulation. Alderman et al. [86] used prompts and rewards to help a patient improve control of inappropriate behaviors through better self-regulation skills.

Medd and Tate [87] carried out a cognitive behavioral program for anger management. The program consisted of 5–8 weekly sessions of individual therapy that included components of stress inoculation, self-verbalization, and cognitive challenging, as well as assertiveness, time out, and self-distraction. Their program was aimed at increasing internalization of self-regulation. The sample in their study was recruited from a rehabilitation unit and was heterogeneous with respect to the diagnosis; none of them had any preinjury, psychiatric, or emotional disturbance [87–89].

## Applications of Cognitive Behavioral Therapy to Emotional Distress in TBI

Individuals with TBI are at greater risk for experiencing increased levels of anxiety as compared to the general population [90]. Research findings have reported difficulties following TBI with *depression* and *anxiety* [91] and *posttraumatic stress disorder* [92]. Emotional difficulties become noticeable in the early stages of recovery, although they may also emerge several years following the injury. However, what is significant is that, similar to the cognitive sequelae, emotional/behavioral sequelae tend to persist over time and have long-lasting effects on a person's functional outcomes, affecting employment, independent living, relationships, and social and leisure activities [91].

The basic premise of CBT is that modification of information processing will lead to changes in emotions and behaviors. CBTs help patients to identify distortions in their thinking and generate more rational interpretations of events [93]. CBT is an evidence-based therapy, and its efficacy in emotional disorders is well established.

In a recent review by the Cochrane Collaboration [94], psychological interventions for individuals with anxiety following TBI were examined. Evidence from case studies demonstrates that CBT reduces anxiety symptomatology in TBI patients. Khan-Bourne and Brown [95] present CBT as a potentially suitable treatment for depression following TBI. Recent studies have evaluated the effectiveness of CBT in treating the emotional and behavioral sequeale of TBI. Bedard et al. [96] delivered 12 weekly group sessions providing insight meditation, breathing exercises, guided visualization, and group discussion. Their study aimed at encouraging patients to adopt a new perspective on life and its difficulties so as to allow a sense of acceptance and to move beyond limiting beliefs. Following therapy, patients reported significant improvements in their quality of life compared to dropout controls. Other researchers report the use of biofeedback-assisted relaxation [97] and mindfulness-based strategies [96].

## Applications to Schizophrenia

This section provides a brief overview of the scope of behavioral and cognitive and metacognitive interventions in patients with schizophrenia. The debate over the scope of cognitive rehabilitation in schizophrenia is over a decade old. Cognitive deficits persist even when symptoms subside and impair the individual's functioning across various spheres of life [98]. Some of the earliest and most convincing evidence came from studies on contingent social and token reinforcement [99]. Deficits in the areas of communication, adaptive functioning, maintaining occupation, and community functioning, though seen in other disorders, are "defining" features in schizophrenia. Cognitive deficits in schizophrenia were increasingly viewed as influencing functional outcome and, hence, targeted for intervention [100]. Green et al. [101] reported that 20–40% of the variance in functional outcome could be explained by composite measures of neurocognition. However, 60–80% of the variance in functional outcome remains unaccounted for. Social cognition refers to the mental operations underlying social interactions, which include processes involved in perceiving, interpreting, and generating responses to the intentions, dispositions, and behaviors of others [102].

Four domains of social cognition, namely emotion processing, theory of mind (ToM), social perception and social knowledge, and attributional style/bias, have been identified. Correlation and structural equation modeling analyses strongly suggest that social cognition serves as a mediating link between neurocognition and community functioning in schizophrenia. Pinkham and Penn [103] found that individuals with schizophrenia demonstrated impaired performance across several domains of neurocognitive and social cognitive functioning (ToM, social knowledge, and emotion perception) as well as interpersonal skills. In addition, among the participants with schizophrenia, social cognition significantly contributed unique variance (an additional 26%) to interpersonal skill beyond that of neurocognition. This pattern was not observed in the nonclinical control sample [103,104].

The Social Cognition and Interaction Training (SCIT) program was developed by Penn et al. (2005). It is a group-based intervention that is delivered weekly over a 6-month period. The main objective of the SCIT is to improve both social cognition and social functioning for individuals with schizophrenia spectrum disorders. The SCIT consists of three components: emotion training, figuring out, and integration. It also addresses metacognitive processes such as jumping to conclusions, cognitive rigidity, and intolerance of ambiguity [105,106]. Another extensive research program that integrates neurocognition with social cognition and macrolevel social skills is integrated psychological therapy (IPT). IPT was developed by Brenner et al. [107]. According to Brenner et al. [108], social dysfunction in schizophrenia is maintained over time due to an interaction between two vicious cycles. In the first cycle, called the type I cycle, deficits in basic cognitive processes diminish higher-order cognitive functioning that are necessary for integrating incoming information. In the type II cycle, cognitive deficits prevent the acquisition of interpersonal coping skills that makes it difficult for patients to cope with social stressors and demands of day-to-day living. As these two cycles interact and reinforce each other, symptoms emerge and social dysfunction ensues. The program is based on the theory that cognitive functioning is organized hierarchically. Cognitive processes such as attention affect other micro- and macrolevel processes such as social skills and coping. IPT is divided into five categories: cognitive differentiation, social perception, verbal communication, social skills, and interpersonal problem solving. The first two components target cognitive deficits, while the other three target social interaction and functioning. The program includes behavioral techniques such as reinforcement, modeling, and role plays as well as interpersonal communication [108,109].

Cognitive Enhancement Therapy (CET) is considered to be a developmental approach to the rehabilitation of schizophrenia patients; the main goal of CET is to facilitate abstracting and social cognition [110,111]. CET is a small group-based program including components such as perspective taking through experiential learning, appraising social contexts, affect regulation, and using reciprocity and shared understanding. These are also believed to be cornerstones of social cognition [112].

The rehabilitation programs offered for patients with schizophrenia have to be focused on core cognitive deficits and social cognition deficits in order to be more holistic and bring about changes in functional outcomes. These are particularly relevant to patients with negative symptoms and social dysfunction.

## The Role of Family

Behavioral disorders are distressing to families, disruptive to therapy, and can jeopardize patient safety. The family has to learn to cope with the behavioral disorders, including the financial as well as psychological "scars" following an injury. These often include the spouse, children, or parents of the patient as well as the treating team. It is, therefore, essential to address the needs of these clients and their families to minimize distress and problems as well as to facilitate and maximize the coping resources and skills of these individuals. The family also plays an important role in both the maintenance of problem behaviors and the development of adaptive functioning.

## Case Illustrations

**Case 1**

Mr. R was a 37-year-old businessman; he had completed a master's degree in engineering and was running his own firm. He was married and lived with his wife, children, and extended family. Prior to the accident, he was described as an intelligent, hardworking person who had taken many initiatives in expanding the family enterprise.

Mr. R met with a road traffic accident while traveling with his family. He suffered severe trauma in the accident, which claimed the life of the driver. Following several months of hospitalization, Mr. R returned home but could not resume his business. A behavioral analysis was carried out to list the target behaviors as well as to understand excesses and deficits. A significant factor that had to be considered in the case of Mr. R was his physical disabilities resulting from the accident. The physical disabilities and complications further interfered with learning and caused impediments and limitations in planning other therapies. At the time of referral, he was in a wheelchair, and due to extensive surgery to the jaw, he could not speak clearly.

The behavioral analysis revealed several behavioral deficits, the most significant being a lack of motivation and interest, low speech output, no attempts at spontaneous speech, and variable eye contact. Mr. R displayed significant disinterest in all his activities and interactions. The lack of interest and motivation had also affected his participation in the cognitive rehabilitation program. The analysis also included assessment of reinforcers, such as social activity. Since Mr. R had significant amotivation, it was planned that positive programming would be used in order to increase his involvement.

In the case of Mr. R, target behaviors were broken down into smaller goals in terms of time and difficulty level. Thus, for example, speech output was further broken down into attempts at starting conversation, speaking in short sentences. He would be verbally reinforced for the attempts. Further topics of interest to him, such as children and sports, were included to facilitate speech. Shaping was used to encourage him to gradually increase the length of time and frequency of eye contact.

These activities were also carried out at home. His wife tried to overdo the tasks given in order to make faster progress. Families must be educated regarding pacing activities, as fatigue can interfere with learning. Further, the patient can become frustrated with repeated pressure to perform, and this may lead to noncompliance. The wife was counseled in this regard.

Therapy extended over 4 months; along with shaping and positive programming, social skills training was given, including initiating and maintaining eye contact and speech. His wife was trained as a cotherapist for the skills practice in addition to the therapist as sessions progressed. Mr. R was also encouraged to interact (even if briefly) with other staff and trainees in the department. Following this intensive training on a daily basis, Mr. R was observed to show more initiative in sessions of physiotherapy and speech therapy. He would greet the therapist at the start of sessions and bid goodbye as he was leaving.

As the family planned to return by the end of 4 months, sessions toward the end were focused on generalization of skills to daily life situations. As the patient was now able to sit for a while and contribute to discussions, albeit for a brief time, it was planned that he would visit their family office for at least 2–3 h initially to build a work habit.

The family left for their home town, and in a telephonic review after 3 months, the patient was reported to have settled into going to the office for one-half of the day. He was also said to be maintaining the level of improvement he had achieved with regard to his social interactions. As the patient had another scheduled surgery for his jaw, further follow-up could not be planned.

## Case 2

Mr. B was a 50-year-old man, married and educated up to a technical training course, and at the time of his accident was working in a factory. He was living with his family, which consisted of his wife and two sons. Mr. B was an idealistic man, described by his family as stubborn, aggressive, and a strict disciplinarian. He was well liked by his fellow workers, but was feared at home for his temper, as he would often get physically and verbally abusive. In a road accident, he suffered injuries to the head, and his speech and mobility were impaired. At the time of referral, Mr. B was entirely dependent on his family for his daily needs. The youngest son was away at school, and his wife and older son would take care of him. The family observed that even a year and half after the TBI, he would be aggressive, spit at others if they tried to interact with him, and would refuse to make eye contact. This included therapists with whom he worked. Mr. B would refuse to cooperate and would scream when requested to comply with any of the tasks. As a consequence of these behavioral problems, the family would withdraw, leading to a vicious cycle of negative reinforcement as well as at times a reversal of roles in which the patient would be rendered powerless due to the family. Mr. B's wife reported feeling depressed and hopeless and helpless about the situation and future.

For Mr. B, differential reinforcement was utilized. A detailed behavioral analysis revealed both excesses such as shouting, spitting, and hitting at times, and deficits such as poor eye contact and not interacting. The disruptive behaviors were placed on an extinction schedule and were ignored or not attended to. The ABC analysis revealed that the triggers for excess behaviors were restriction and not paying attention; at times, it was also an effort to communicate his anger toward his son. The patient's son was one of the caregivers, and it was noted that he was inadvertently using too much of restriction on the patient. This would lead to the patient shouting till he was let free. This would frustrate him and lead to noncompliance. Positive and socially appropriate behaviors such as greeting visitors and not abusing family members were rewarded with social reinforcements of verbal praise that the patient appreciated. Another behavioral strategy employed for developing social behaviors was that of shaping. For the time period when he kept eye contact he would be rewarded, and this time was gradually increased. Time out in the form of the therapist leaving the room for brief periods contingent on shouting was also employed. This helped in reducing disruptive behaviors during sessions. Shaping and positive reinforcements were also used to increase self-help tasks such as assisting caregivers while dressing and eating.

Mr. B's referral was also due to the fact that he was noncompliant with cognitive retraining. Following the sessions of behavior therapy, he was able to sit for at least 20 min during the session. During this session, he would be compliant and would not shout or spit. He was socially reinforced for this. Similarly, the family was counseled to practice the use of positive reinforcements for desirable behaviors. The wife was also counseled individually as she had faced considerable stress in caregiving. This would lead to her becoming angry and affecting the patient.

The patient was followed up for about 6 months, after which time they moved back to their home. He was reported to be maintaining improvements made in sessions.

## Conclusions

* TBI leads to significant behavioral, cognitive, emotional, and social consequences for the individual and family.
* Behavioral methods have wide utility in the rehabilitation of individuals with TBI for problems such as aggressive, inappropriate behaviors, and social and communication skills. Strategies based on operant conditioning include reinforcement contingencies, response cost, time out, modeling, role plays, and rehearsal with feedback.
* The improvement of executive functions is an important area in which cognitive behavioral principles are applied and involves self-awareness and knowledge, self-regulation, and information processing.
* Incorporating behavioral, cognitive, and social interventions would enhance the efficacy of neuro rehabilitation for TBI.
* One of the major limitations of behavior and cognitive behavior therapies has been a lack of controlled studies.

## References

[1] Schoenhuber, R., & Gentilini, M. (1988). Anxiety and depression after mild head injury: A case control study. *Journal of Neurology, Neurosurgery, and Psychiatry,* *51*, 722–724.
[2] Rosenthal, M., & Bond, M. R. (1990). Behavioral and psychaitric sequelae. In M. Rosenthal., E. R. Griffith, M. R. Bond, & J. D. Miller (Eds.), *Rehabilitation of the adult and child with traumatic brain injury* (pp. 179–192) ((2nd ed.)). Philadephia: Dav.
[3] Cicerone, K. D., Dahlberg, C., Malec, J. F., Langenbahn, D. M., Felicetti, T., Kneipp, S., et al. (2005). Evidence based cognitive rehabilitation: Updated review of the literature from 1998 through 2002. *Archives of Physical Medicine and Rehabilitation, 86,* 1681–1692.
[4] Horton, A. M., Jr. (1979). Behavioral neuropsychology: Rationale and research. *Clinical Neuropsychology, 1,* 20–23.
[5] Wood, R. L., & Burgess, P., (1988). The psychological management of behavior disorders following brain injury. In I. Fussey & G. M. Muir (Eds.) Rehabilitation of the severely brain injured adult: a practical approach. Croom Helm (pp. 43–68).
[6] Wood, R. L., & Fussey, I. (Eds.). (1991). *Cognitive rehabilitation in perspective.* London: Taylor and Francis.

[7] Wood, R. L. (1992). A neurobehavioral approach to brain injury in rehabilitation. In N von Steinbüchel, D. Y von Cramon, & E Pöppel (Eds.), *Neuropsychological rehabilitation* (pp. 51–54). Berlin: Springer-Verlag.

[8] Goldstein, G., & Ruthven, L. (1983). *Rehabilitation of the brain injured individual*. New York: Plenum Press.

[9] Horton, A. M., & Barrett, D. (1988). Neurological assessment and behavior therapy: New directions in head trauma rehabilitation. *Journal of Head Trauma Rehabilitattion, 3*(1), 57–64.

[10] McGlynn, S. M. (1990). Behavioral approaches to neuropsychological rehabilitation. *Psychological Bulletin, 108*, 420–441.

[11] Lawson-Kerr, K., Smith, P., & Beck, D. (1991). Behavioral neuropsychology, past, presents direction with organically based mood/affective disorders. *Neuropsychology Review, 2*(1), 65–107.

[12] Horton, A. M., & Puente, A. (1986). Behavioral neuropsychology with children. In G. Hynd & J. Ogrutz (Eds.), *Child neuropsychology* (Vol 2). New York: Academic Press.

[13] Horton, A. M., Jr., & Sautter, S. W. (1986). Behavioral neuro-psychology. In D. Wedding, A. M. Horton Jr., & J. S. Webster (Eds.), *Handbook of clinical and behavioral neuropsychology* (pp. 259–277). New York: Springer.

[14] Horton, A. M., Jr., Wedding, D., & Phay, A. (1981). Current perspectives on assessment and therapy for the brain damaged individual. In C. J. Golden, S. S. A Caparras, F. D. Strider, & B. Graber (Eds.), *Applied techniques in behavioral medicine* (pp. 59–86). New York: Grune and Stratton.

[15] Fordyce, W. E. (1982). Psychological assessment and management. In F. J Kotte, G. K. Stillwell, & J. F. Lehemann (Eds.), *Kruser's handbook of physical medicine and rehabilitation* (pp. 124–150). Philadelphia: W.B. Saunders.

[16] Horton, A. M., Jr., & Howe, N. R. (1981). Behavioural treatment of the traumatically brain injured: A case study. *Perceptual and Motor Skills, 53*, 349–350.

[17] Ben-Yishay, Y., & Gold, J. (1990). Therapeutic milieu approach to neurorehabilittaion. In R. L. Wood. (Ed.), *Neurobehavioral sequelae of traumatic brain injury* (pp. 195–215). London: Taylor and Francis.

[18] Serno, X. (1987). Operant procedures and neuropsychological rehabilitation. In M. J. Meier, A. L. Benton, & L. Diller (Eds.), *Neuropsychological rehabilitation* (pp. 132–162). Edinburgh: Churchill Livingstone.

[19] Ylvisaker, M., Turkstra, L. S., & Coelho, C. (2005). Behavioral and social interventions for individuals with traumatic brain injury: A summary of the research with clinical implications. *Seminars in Speech and Language, 26*(4), 256–267.

[20] Ylvisaker, M., Turkstra, L., Coehlo, C., Yorkston, K., Kennedy, M., Sohlberg, M. M., et al. (2008). Behavioural interventions for children and adults with behaviour disorders after TBI: A systematic review of the evidence. *Brain Injury, 21*(8), 769–805.

[21] Prigatano, G. (1986). *Neuropsychological rehabilitation after brain injury*. Baltimore, MD: John Hopkins University Press.

[22] Glasgow, R. E., Zeiss, R. A., Barrera, M., Jr., & Lewinsohn, P. M. (1977). Case studies on remediating brain damage deficits in brain damaged individuals. *Journal of Clinical Psychology, 33*, 1049–1054.

[23] Godoy, J. F. (1990). Estrategias de intervencixn en neuropsicologia. I Jornadas Nacionales de Neuropsicologia Clinica Funciones Cerebrales. Almeria.

[24] Gracey, F. (2002). Mood and affective problems after traumatic brain injury. *ACNR, 2*(3), 18–20.

[25] Levin, H. S., Benton, A. L., & Grossman, R. G. (1982). *Neurobehavioral consequences of closed head injury*. New York: Oxford University Press.

[26] Alderman, N., & Burgess, P. (1994). A comparison of treatment methods for behavior disorder following herpes simplex encephalitis. *Neuropsychological Rehabilitation, 4,* 31–48.

[27] Cohen, R. E. (1986). Behavioral treatment of incontinence in a profoundly neurologically impaired adult. *Archives of Physical Medicine and Rehabilitation, 67,* 883–884.

[28] Hollon, T. H. (1973). Behavior modification in a community hospital rehabilitation unit. *Archives of Physical Medicine and Rehabilitation, 54,* 65–72.

[29] Jacobs, H. E., Lynch, M., Cornick, J., & Slifer, K. (1986). Behavior management of aggressive sequeale after Reye's syndrome. *Archives of Physical Medicine and Rehabilitation, 67,* 558–563.

[30] Turner, J. M., Green, G., & Braunling-McMorrow, D. (1990). Differential reinforcement of low rates of responding (DRL) to reduce dysfunctional social behaviors of a head injured man. *Behavioral Residential Treatment, 5,* 15–27.

[31] Foxx, R. M., & Azrin, N. H. (1972). Restitution: A method of eliminating aggressive–disruptive behavior of retarded brain damaged patients. *Behavior Research and Therapy, 10,* 15–27.

[32] Wood, R. L. (1987). *Brain injury rehabilitation: A neurobehavioral approach.* Rockville, MD: Aspen Publishers.

[33] Burgess, P. W., & Alderman, N. (1990). Rehabilitation of dyscontrol syndromes following frontal lobe damage: A cognitive neuropsychological approach. In R. L Wood, & I. Fussey (Eds.), *Cognitive rehabilitation in perspective* (pp. 183–203). London: Taylor and Francis.

[34] Wood, R. L, & Eames, P. (1981). Application of behaviour modification in the rehabilitation of traumatically brain-injured patients. In G. Davey (Ed.), *Applications of conditioning theory* (pp. 81–101). London: Methuen.

[35] Alderman, N., & Knight, C. (1997). The effectiveness of DRL in the management and treatment of severe behaviour disorders following brain injury. *Brain Injury, 11*(79), 101.

[36] Hegel, M. T., & Ferguson, R. J. (2000). Differential reinforcement of other behavior (DRO) to reduce aggressive behavior following traumatic brain injury. *Behavior Modification, 24*(1), 94–101.

[37] Becker, M. E., & Vakil, E. (1993). Behavioral psychotherapy in the frontal lobe injured patient in an outpatient setting. *Brain Injury, 7*(6), 15–23.

[38] Aeschleman, S. R., & Imes, C. (1999). Stress inoculation training for impulsive behaviors in adults with traumatic brain injury. *Journal of Rational-Emotive and Cognitive Behavior Therapy, 17,* 51–65.

[39] Uswatte, G., & Taub, E. (1999). In D. T. Stuss, C. Winocur, & I. H. Robertson (Eds.), *Cognitive rehabilitation* (pp. 215–230). Cambridge: Cambridge University Press.

[40] Pulvermuller, F., Neininger, B., Elbert, T., Mohr, B., Rockstroh, B., Koebbel, P., et al. (2001). Constraint-induced therapy of chronic aphasia after stroke. *Stroke, 32*(7), 1621–1626.

[41] Amato, A., Hermseyer, C. A., & Kleinman, K. M. (1983). Use of electromyography feedback to increase inhibitory control of spastic muscles. *Physical Therapy, 53,* 1063–1066.

[42] Brundy, J., Korein, J., Grynbaum, B. B., Belandres, P. V., & Giantusos, J. G. (1979). Helping hemiparetics to help themselves: Sensory feedback therapy. *Journal of the American Medical Association, 241,* 814–818.

[43] Brundy, J., Korein, J., Grynbaum, B. B., & Sachs- Frankel, G. (1977). Sensory feedback therapy in patients with brain insult. *Scandinavian Journal of Rehabilitation Medicine, 9,* 155–163.

[44] Frazier, L. M. (1980). Biofeedback in Coma rehabilitation: A case study. *American Journal of Clinical Feedback, 3,* 48–54.

[45] Sterman, M. B., Wyrwicka, W., & Roth, S. R. (1969). Electrophysiological correlates and neural substrates of alimentary behavior in the cat. *Annals of New York Academy of Science*, *157*, 723–739.

[46] Laibow, R. (1999). Medical applications of neurobiofeedback. In J. R. Evans, & A. Abarbanel (Eds.), *Introduction to quantitative EEG and neurofeedback*. New York: Academic Press.

[47] Thatcher, R. W. (2000). EEG operant conditioning (biofeedback) and traumatic brain injury. *Clinical Electroencephalography*, *31*(1), 38–44.

[48] Byers, A. P. (1995). Neurofeedback therapy for a mild head injury. *Journal of Neurotherapy*, *1*(1), 22–37.

[49] Hoffman, D. A., Stockdale, S., & Van Egren, L. (1996). Symptom changes in the treatment of mild traumatic brain injury using EEG neurofeedback (Abstract). *Clinical Electroencephalography*, *27*(3), 164.

[50] Keller, I. (2001). Neurofeedback therapy of attention deficits in patients with traumatic brain injury. *Journal of Neurotherapy*, *5*(1–2), 19–32.

[51] Walker, J. E., Norman, C. A., & Weber, R. K. (2002). Impact of qEEG-guided coherence training for patients with mild closed head injury. *Journal of Neurotherapy*, *6*(2), 31–33.

[52] Sterman, M. B. (2000). Basic concepts and clinical findings in seizure disorders with EEG operant conditioning. *Clinical Electroencephalography*, *31*(1), 45–55.

[53] Thornton, K. (2002). Rehabilitation of memory functioning with EEG. Biofeedback. *NeuroRehabilitation*, *17*(1), 69.

[54] Kennedy, M. R. T., & Coelho, C. (2005). Self-regulation after traumatic brain injury: A framework for intervention of memory and problem solving. *Seminars in Speech and Language*, *26*(4), 242–255.

[55] Kennedy, M. R. T., & Turkstra, L. (2006). Group intervention studies in the cognitive rehabilitation of individuals with traumatic brain injury: Challenges faced by researchers. *Neuropsychology Review*, *16*, 151–159.

[56] Kennedy, M. R. T, Coelho, C., Turkstra, L., Ylvisaker, M., Sohlberg, M. M., Yorkston, K., et al. (2008). Intervention for executive functions after traumatic brain injury: A systematic review, meta-analysis and clinical recommendations. *Neuropsychological Rehabilitation*, 1–43.

[57] Wells, A. (1997). *Cognitive therapy of anxiety disorders: A practice manual and conceptual guide*. Chichester, UK: Wiley.

[58] Ben-Yishay, Y., & Diller, L. (1983). Cognitive remediation. In M. Rosenthal, E. R. Griffith, M. R. Bond, & J. D. Miller (Eds.), *Rehabilitation of the head-injured adult* (pp. 367–379). Philadelphia: F.A. Davis.

[59] Goldstein, F. C., & Levin, H. S. (1987). Disorders of reasoning and problem-solving ability. In M. Meier, A. Benton, & L. Diller (Eds.), *Neuropsychological rehabilitation*. London: Taylor and Francis.

[60] Baddeley, A., & Wilson, B. (1988). Frontal amnesia and the dysexecutive syndrome. *Brain and Cognition*, *7*, 212–230.

[61] Luria, A. R. (1963). *Restoration of function after brain injury*. Oxford: Pergamon Press.

[62] Luria, A. R. (1966). *Human brain and psychological processes*. New York: Harper and Row.

[63] Bruner, J. S., Goodnow, J. J., & Austin, G. A. (1956). *A study of thinking*. New York: Wiley.

[64] D'Zurilla, T. J., & Goldfried, M. R. (1971). Problem solving and behavior modification. *Journal of Abnormal Psychology*, *78*, 107–126.

[65] D'Zurilla, T. J., & Nezu, A. M. (1982). Social problem-solving in adults. In P. C. (1982). Kendall (Ed.), *Advances in cognitive behavioral research and therapy Vol. 1*, (pp. 201–274). New York: Acedemic Press.

[66] D'Zurilla, T. J, & Nezu, A. M. (2001). Problem solving therapies. In K. S. Dobson (Ed.), *Handbook of cognitive behavioral therapies* (pp. 211–245) (2nd ed.). New York: Guilford Press.

[67] Rath, J. F., Simon, D., Langenbahn, D. M., Sherr, R. L., & Diller, L. (2003). Group treatment of problem-solving deficits in outpatients with traumatic brain injury: A randomised outcome study. *Neuropsychological Rehabilitation, 13*(4), 461–488.

[68] D'Zurilla, T. J., & Maydeu-Olivares, A. (1995). Conceptual and methodological issues in social problem-solving assessment. *Behavior Therapy, 26,* 409–432.

[69] Winkler, D., Unsworth, C., & Sloan, S. (2006). Factors that lead to successful community integration following severe traumatic brain injury. *Journal of Head Trauma Rehabilitation, 21,* 8–21.

[70] Fasotti, L., Kovacs, F., Eling, P. A. T. M., & Brouwer, W. H. (2000). Time pressure management as a compensatory strategy training after closed head injury. *Neuropsychological Rehabilitation, 10,* 47–65.

[71] Cicerone, K. D., & Giacino, J. T. (1992). Remediation of executive function deficits after traumatic brain injury. *NeuroRehabilitation, 2,* 12–22.

[72] Suzman, K. B., Morris, R. D., Morris, M. K., & Milan, M. A. (1997). Cognitive-behavioral remediation of problem solving deficits in children with acquired brain injury. *Journal of Behavioral Therapy and Experimental Psychiatry, 28,* 203–212.

[73] Burke, W. H., Zencius, A. H., Wesolowski, M. D., & Doubleday, F. (1991). Improving executive function disorders in brain-injured clients. *Brain Injury, 5,* 241–252.

[74] Levine, B., Robertson, I., Clare, L., Carter, G., Hong, J., Wilson, B. A., et al. (2000). Rehabilitation of executive functioning: An experimental-clinical validation of goal management training. *Journal of the International Neuropsychological Society, 6,* 299–312.

[75] Webb, P. M., & Gluecauf, R. L. (1994). The effects of direct involvement in goal setting on rehabilitation outcome for persons with traumatic brain injuries. *Rehabilitation Psychology, 39,* 179–188.

[76] Von Cramon, D. Y., Matthes-von Cramon, G, & Mai, N. (1991). Problem solving deficits in brain-injured patients: A therapeutic approach. *Neuropsychological Rehabilitation, 1,* 45–64.

[77] Cicerone, K. D., & Wood, J. C. (1987). Planning disorder after closed head injury: A case study. *Archives of Physical Medicine and Rehabilitation, 68,* 111–115.

[78] Delazer, M., Bodner, T., & Benke, T. (1998). Rehabilitation of arithmetical test problem solving. *Neuropsychological Rehabilitation, 8,* 401–412.

[79] Fox, R. M., Marchand-Martella., N. E., Martella, R. C., Braunling-McMorrow, D., & McMorrow, M. J. (1988). Teaching a problem-solving strategy to closed head-injured adults. *Behavioral Interventions, 3*(3), 194–210.

[80] Marshall, R. C., Karow, C. M., Morelli, C. A., Iden, K. K., Dixon, J., & Cranfill, T. B. (2004). Effects of interactive strategy modeling training on problem-solving by persons with traumatic brain injury. *Aphasiology, 18,* 650–673.

[81] Manly, T., Hawkins, K., Evans, J., Woldt, K., & Robertson, I. H. (2001). Rehabilitation ofexecutive function: Facilitation of effective goal management on complex tasks using periodic auditory alerts. *Neuropsychologia, 40,* 271–281.

[82] Turkstra, L. S., & Flora, T. L. (2002). Compensating for executive function impairments after TBI: A single case study of functional intervention. *Journal of Communication Disorders, 35*(6), 467–482.

[83] Stablum, F., Umilta, C., Mogentale, C., Carlan, M., & Guerrini, C. (2000). Rehabilitation of executive deficits in closed head injury and anterior communicating artery aneurysm patients. *Psychological Research, 63,* 265–278.

[84] Cicerone, K., Levin, H., Malec, J., Stuss, D., & Whyte, J. (2006). Cognitive rehabilitation interventions for executive function: Moving from bench to bedside in patients with rraumatic brain injury. *Journal of Cognitive Neuroscience*, *18*(7), 1212–1222.

[85] Fasotti, L. (2003). Executive function retraining (2nd ed.). In J. Grafman & I. H. Robertson (Eds.), *Handbook of neuropsychology Vol. 9*, (pp. 67–78). New York: Elsiever Science.

[86] Alderman, N., Fry, R. K., & Youngson, H. A. (1995). Improvement of self monitoring skills, reduction of behavior disturbance and the dysexecutive syndrome: Comparison of response cost and a new program of self-monitoring training. *Neuropsychological Rehabilitation*, *5*, 193–221.

[87] Medd, J., & Tate, R. L. (2000). Evaluation of an anger management therapy program following acquired brain injury: A preliminary study. *Neuropsychological Rehabilitation*, *10*, 185–201.

[88] Ownsworth, T. L., & McFarland, K. (1999). Memory remediation in the long term acquired brain injury: Two approaches to diary training. *Brain Injury*, *13*, 605–626.

[89] Owns worth, T. L., McFarland, K., & Young Rmc, D. (2000). Self awareness and psychosocial functioning following acquired brain injury: An evaluation of a group support program. *Neuropsychological Rehabilitation*, *10*, 465–484.

[90] Hiott, D. W., & Labbate, L. (2002). Anxiety disorders associated with traumatic brain injuries. *NeuroRehabilitation*, *17*, 345–355.

[91] Kersel, D. A., Marsh, N. V., Havill, J. H., & Sleigh, J. W. (2001). PsychosocialFunctioning during the year following severe traumatic brain injury. *Brain Injury*, *15*(8), 683.

[92] Bryant, R. A., Marosszeky, J. E., Crooks, J., Baguley, I. J., & Gurka, J. A. (2001). Posttraumatic stress disorder and psychosocial functioning after severe traumatic brain injury. *Journal of Nervous and Mental Disease*, *189*(2), 109–113.

[93] Alderman, N. (2003). Contemporary approaches to the management of irritability and aggression following traumatic brain injury. *Neuropsychological Rehabilitation*, *13*, 211–240.

[94] Soo, C., & Tate, R. (2007). Psychological treatment for anxiety in people with traumatic brain injury. *Cochrane Database of Systematic Reviews*, *3*, CD005239. doi:10.1002/14651858.CD005239.pub2.

[95] Khan-Bourne, N., & Brown, R. G. (2003). Cognitive behavior therapy for the treatment of depression in individuals with brain injury. *Neuropsychological Rehabilitation*, *13*(1–2), 89–107.

[96] Bedard, M., Felteau, M., Mazmanian, D., Fedyk, K., Klein, R., Richardson, J., et al. (2003). Pilot evaluation of a mindfulness-based intervention to improve quality of life among individuals who sustained traumatic brain injuries. *Disability and Rehabilitation*, *25*, 722–723.

[97] Ackerman, R. J. (2004). Applied psychophysiology, clinical biofeedback, and rehabilitation neuropsychology: A case study – mild traumatic brain injury and posttraumatic stress disorder. *Physical Medicine and Rehabilitation Clinics of North America*, *4*(15), 919–931.

[98] Spring, B., & Ravdin, L. (1992). Cognitive remediation in schizophrenia: Should we attempt it in schizophrenia. *Schizophrenia Bulletin*, *18*(1), 15–20.

[99] Meichenbaum, D. H. (1969). The effects of instructions and reinforcement on thinking and language behavior of schizophrenics. *Behavior Research and Therapy*, *7*, 101–114.

[100] Green, M. F., & Nuechterlein, K. H. (1999). Should schizophrenia be treated as a neurocognitive disorder? *Schizophrenia Bulletin, 25*, 309–318.

[101] Green, M. F., Kern, R. S., Braff, D. L., & Mintz, J. (2000). Neurocognitive deficits & functional outcome in schizophrenia: Are we measuring the right stuff? *Schizophrenia Bulletin, 26*, 119–136.

[102] Green, M. F., Olivier, B., Crawley, J. N., Penn, D. L., & Silverstein, S. (2005). Social cognition in schizophrenia: Recommendations from the MATRICS new approaches conference. *Schizophrenia Bulletin, 31*, 882–887.

[103] Pinkham, A. E., & Penn, D. L. (2006). Neurocognitive & social cognitive predictors of interpersonal skill in schizophrenia. *Psychiatry Research, 143*, 167–178.

[104] Penn, D. L., & Mueser, K. T. (1996). Research update on the psychosocial treatment of schizophrenia. *American Journal of Psychiatry, 153*, 607–617.

[105] Penn, D. L., Roberts, D., Munt, E. D., Silverstein, E., & Sheitman, B. (2005). A pilot study of social cognition and interaction training (SCIT) for schizophrenia. *Schizophrenia Research, 80*, 357–359.

[106] Penn, D. L., Roberts, D. L., Combs, D., & Sterne, A. (2007). Best practices: The development of the social cognition and interaction training program for schizophrenia spectrum disorders. *Psychiatric Services, 58*, 449–451.

[107] Brenner, H. D., Hodel, B., & Roder, V. (1990). Integrated cognitive and behavioral interventions in treatment of schizophrenia. *Psychosocial Rehabilitation Journal, 13*, 41–43.

[108] Brenner, H. D., Hodel, B., Roder, V., & Corrigan, P. (1992). Integrated psychological therapy for schizophrenic patients (IPT): Basic assumptions, current status and future directions. In F. P. Ferrero, A. E. Haynal, & N. Sartorius (Eds.), *Schizophrenia and affective psychoses: Nosology in contemporary psychiatry* (pp. 201–209). London: John Libbey.

[109] Brenner, H. D., Roder, V., Hodel, B., Kienzle, N., Reed, D., & Liberman, R. P. (1994). *Integrated psychological therapy for schizophrenic patients*. Toronto, Canada: Hogrefe & Huber.

[110] Hogarty, Q. E., & Flesher, S. (1999). Practice principles of cognitive enhancement therapy for schizophrenia. *Schizophrenia Bulletin, 25*(4), 693–708.

[111] Gerard, E., Hogarty, G. E., Greenwals, D. P., & Eack, S. M. (2006). Durability and mechanism of effects of cognitive enhancement therapy. *Psychiatric Services, 57*, 1751–1757.

[112] Twamley, E. W., Jeste, D. V., & Bellack, A. B. (2003). A review of cognitive training in schizophrenia. *Schizophrenia Bulletin, 29*(2), 359–382.

# 6 Neuropsychological Rehabilitation in Neurological Conditions: A Circuitry Approach

## J. Keshav Kumar

Associate Professor and Consultant Neuropsychologist, Neuropsychology Unit, Department of Clinical Psychology, National Institute of Mental Health and Neurosciences (NIMHANS), Bangalore, Karnataka, India

Advances in medical sciences have increased the chances of survival after acquired brain damage for patients with neurological conditions such as stroke and traumatic brain injury. Often they are left with physical, psychological, and cognitive disabilities. These disabilities impede their return to employment and reintegration into society. Cognitive deficits include impairments in attention, concentration, learning and memory, executive functions, and personality changes in the form of increased irritability, poor motivation, apathy, and depression. Survivors of head injury present with an array of symptoms including headache, dizziness, vertigo, tinnitus, hearing loss, blurred vision, diplopia, convergence insufficiency, light and noise sensitivity, diminished taste and smell, irritability, anxiety, depression, personality change, fatigue, sleep disturbance, and decreased appetite and libido. In addition, they have deficits in the cognitive realm such as impairments of attention, speed of processing, executive functions, memory, and visuoperceptual skills. Personality change is also reported [1,2].

Cognitive deficits are the most debilitating sequelae following neurological conditions and are often protracted. All cognitive functions are not uniformly affected; some cognitive functions may remain intact, while other functions may be impaired [3]. Cognitive deficits have an impact on the patient's ability to return to employment and reintegration into society, and they are often a primary cause for loss of productive employment [4]. A number of studies have demonstrated that neuropsychological rehabilitation is efficacious in improving cognitive deficits following acquired brain injury. Several studies indicating improvement of cognitive deficits in the domains of attention, executive functions, learning and memory, and behavioral problems following traumatic brain injury have been reported [5]; however, the primary focus of neuropsychological rehabilitation has been on head-injured patients.

Cognitive deficits have been demonstrated in other neurological conditions such as stroke and encephalitis and are evident in both acute and later phases of the

Neuropsychological Rehabilitation-Principles and Applications.
DOI: http://dx.doi.org/10.1016/B978-0-12-416046-0.00006-7

illness. In encephalitis, there is an inflammation in the brain parenchyma resulting from a virus or bacteria. At the acute stage, there is documentation of mental changes and the cognitive deficits following encephalitis beyond the acute phase of illness. Infectious diseases such as herpes simplex encephalitis results in severe memory deficits [6,7] resulting from bilateral damage to the temporal lobes [8]. The memory deficits seen in herpes simplex encephalitis include deficits in verbal memory, visual memory, and personality changes in the form of behavioral disturbances such as euphoria, mania, aggression, irritability, and depressive mood [9].

Similar cognitive deficits are experienced in patients with stroke. Recent studies suggest that about 64% of individuals suffering from stroke have cognitive deficits, and a substantial portion of them develop dementia [10–12]. The cognitive deficits resulting from stroke are referred to as "vascular cognitive impairments" (VCI). About 50% of patients suffering from VCI develop dementia [13].

# Neuropsychological Rehabilitation

Neuropsychological rehabilitation involves procedures aimed at (1) restoring defective cognitive abilities through direct retraining and (2) teaching compensatory strategies to circumvent the impaired cognitive abilities. The aim of the restorative approach is to enhance neural plasticity as well as to increase some amount of functional ability. A number of studies have demonstrated improvement in cognitive functions in the domains of attention, executive function, and memory [5].

## Attention Rehabilitation

Studies aimed at attention rehabilitation have used methods such as computer programs that require the patient to respond to particular stimuli as rapidly as possible [14,15]. Researchers have developed a computerized program [16] in which tasks with increasing complexity are presented in a hierarchical fashion; improvements have been found in visual and auditory reaction time as well as improvement in verbal IQ on the Wechsler adult intelligence scale (WAIS). Other methods include reaction time tasks, various visuomotor tasks, visual search tasks [17], scanning moving symbols on a computer screen [18], and video games [19] to enhance sustained attention and speed of processing. These studies have found gradual and significant increases in the number of correct responses after the training.

## Memory Rehabilitation

The earliest record of rehabilitation of memory involves the use of mnemonic strategies that demonstrated improvement. Patients were trained to couple a list of objects with a predetermined series of numbers [20]. Visual imagery has been used to enhance paired associate learning and face–name learning. Imagery was found to be useful in memory training [21–23]. A combination of visual imagery, mnemonic techniques, and training on organizational strategies for 1 h a week over 3 months resulted in 50% improvement in memory performance [24]. Computer-based rehabilitation has also been used to ameliorate memory deficits. Glisky et al. [25] used vanishing cues to teach simple computer commands or vocabulary to head-injured patients. The patients were able to learn and remember simple computer commands and maintain the improvement on the follow-up assessment after 9 months. External memory aids or prosthetic devices have been used to augment memory in head-injured patients. This includes use of memory diaries, writing on calendars, digital alarms, and use of PDA and cell phones. Training on attention using a hierarchical model with five levels of attention including focused, sustained, selective, alternating, and divided attention has been found to be useful in enhancing working memory, and it is associated with improvement in anterograde memory functions [26].

### Executive Functions Training

There are very few studies on rehabilitation of executive functions in head-injured patients. Cicerone and Wood [27] trained head-injured patients on Tower of London to enhance executive functions and problem-solving ability. Brainstorming designs by breaking problems into steps such as generating alternatives, simultaneous analysis of information from multiple sources, and drawing inferences based on available information have also been used to enhance problem-solving ability [28].

### Multimodal Interventions

Multimodal interventions to address impairment in multiple cognitive domains such as attention, memory, and problem solving have been employed. The domains are addressed sequentially or concurrently. Head-injured individuals trained on attention, memory, and problem-solving abilities on computer- versus noncomputer-assisted intervention showed significant improvement on neuropsychological measures following intervention; however, no difference was evident between computer- versus noncomputer-based intervention [29,30]. Large numbers of studies on rehabilitation of cognitive deficits have serious limitation in terms of small samples; some had no control groups, and some had poor generalization to everyday function.

## Neuropsychological Rehabilitation in India

The neuropsychological rehabilitation program at the Neuropsychology Unit, Department of Clinical Psychology, National Institute of Mental Health and Neurosciences (NIMHANS) was started in 1986. The rehabilitation program initially targeted improvement of cognitive deficits resulting from traumatic brain injury. Over the years, several rehabilitation programs for neurological and psychiatric conditions have been developed by the Neuropsychological Unit. Rehabilitation programs are individually tailored, customized for patients following a comprehensive neuropsychological assessment. The rehabilitation programs cater to both urban and rural Indian populations from different socioeconomic strata. It is challenging to develop a cost-effective rehabilitation program using material that is easily available to every patient. Several studies have been conducted to rehabilitate cognitive deficits in head-injured patients. Nag-Arulmani and Rao [31] improved attention functions; the training addressed focused, sustained, and divided attention on four head-injured patients. Remediation was done for 1 month, with each session lasting 45 min. They found improvement on serial processing in two patients and parallel processing in two patients. Neuropsychological deficits did not improve; however, symptom intensity and behavioral functions improved significantly in three out of the four patients. The findings indicated that attention retraining and attention improvement facilitates symptom reduction. However, the limitation of this study is that the sample size was small.

Remediation of memory functions, particularly increasing the automaticity of encoding processes, was attempted in another study [32]. The focus was to train encoding of contextual cues such as frequency and temporal and spatial aspects of memory, which would augment memory function as a whole. The treatment group improved on memory functions as well as other neuropsychological functions as compared to the no-treatment control group.

A comprehensive multimodal approach to improve cognitive function was developed for patients with traumatic brain injury [33] (Kumar et al., unpublished thesis). The sample comprised of 20 patients who received neuropsychological rehabilitation on a daily basis for 30 sessions and were compared with 20 head-injured patients who did not receive neuropsychological rehabilitation. The patients were included into the study 3 months after head injury to allow spontaneous recovery to occur. The rehabilitation program addressed cognitive domains including attention, executive function such as response inhibition, mental flexibility, verbal fluency, divided attention, planning, working memory, and organization. Encoding strategies such as temporal, spatial, and frequency organization of the material to be learned were used to improve memory. The rehabilitation program was developed to enhance the functioning of the fronto-subcortical circuitry. On postassessment, the treatment group showed improvement on all neuropsychological parameters including attention, executive function, and memory. In addition, there was significant symptom reduction and increased subjective well-being on the functional outcome measures. This was also corroborated by relatives of the patients, suggesting generalization to everyday functioning as well. This approach has been extended to other acquired brain damage such as stroke and viral encephalitis, and the results have been promising [34]. Based on this study, a neuropsychological rehabilitation model was developed and has been used.

Encouraged by the results of the hospital-based neuropsychological rehabilitation program, a cost-effective home-based neuropsychological rehabilitation has been developed by the neuropsychological unit to reach out to the masses. The home-based program consists of weekly modules (5 weeks) comprising of paper-and-pencil tasks to improve attention, working memory, response inhibition, and long-term memory. The tasks are performed at home by the patient. The patient's performance is reviewed once a week, and the tasks for the next week are provided. At the end of 5 weeks, mild-to-moderate head-injured patients improved on the tasks, on neuropsychological functions, on EEG parameters, and their symptoms had reduced and everyday functioning improved.

Computerized rehabilitation programs have also been used for retraining of traumatic brain-injured patients. In the initial studies, simple and choice reaction time paradigms were used to improve serial processing of visual information. The span of apprehension tasks was used to improve parallel information processing. The stimuli were Arabic digits presented on the computer. Stimulus duration was tied to the speed and accuracy of the patient's response. In every subsequent trial, the stimulus duration decreased by 1 ms if the response was accurate in the previous trial. Feedback was given to the patient for correct responses. Daily practice was given over 4–6 weeks, with the task difficulty being increased as the patient improved. Task-specific improvement and improvement of neuropsychological functions occurred. Generalization of improvement to everyday life occurred modestly [35]. In another computer-based program, various cognitive functions such as visual attention, visual perception, working memory, mental control, verbal processing, and response inhibition were targeted. The program involves presentation of stimulus material on a computer monitor with increasing difficulty levels. Performance is evaluated mainly in terms of the accuracy of the response of the subject. The exposure time, intertrial duration, and complexity of the stimuli are controlled, being set to increase in a graded manner so as to increase the efficiency of detection/processing by the subject. This program is found to be efficacious in rehabilitation of cognitive deficits following head injury [36].

Similar to the international studies, rehabilitation programs focusing on strategy training with increasing complexity and with tasks presented in a hierarchical fashion have shown improvement in the trained domain. Training provided in multiple domains has been found to be effective.

Despite a proliferation of studies demonstrating the efficacy of neuropsychological rehabilitation, with a few theoretical models to follow, there is no consensuses on how these therapies actually work, and there are no agreed-on guidelines as to how to rehabilitate cognitive deficits resulting from acquired brain damage. Researchers [37] have argued that the focus of rehabilitation should address both compensation as a mechanism of recovery and recovery of neuropsychological functions in full or in part, with the aim of enabling individuals with acquired brain damage to learn not only alternate ways of functioning but also to perform cognitive activities prior to brain injury. The rationale for rehabilitation [37] is based on the notion that practice on carefully selected tasks promotes recovery of the damaged neural circuits and restores functions in the impaired cognitive processes themselves. The tasks mediated by those circuits are then performed in a way similar to nonbrain-damaged individuals [4,37,38]. There are several studies employing various methods of cognitive retraining with varying degrees of improvement reported. However, the mechanism of how these therapies work is still unclear.

Clarity regarding the mechanism of recovery brought about by these retraining programs would help to refine and develop scientifically sound rehabilitation programs for head-injured individuals. The improvement noticed in studies targeting multiple components of cognition also show generalizability to day-to-day functioning. One possible reason for this could be that these rehabilitation programs offer training using different stimulus modalities at increasing levels of complexity and response demands. These include the use of strategies such as organization, verbal naming, mnemonics, and self-regulation such as self-instruction and self-questioning. The use of such strategies can be subsumed under executive functions.

The executive functions are conceptualized as the central executive of the information-processing system, which directs attention and monitors activity, coordination, and integration of information and activity [39]. Executive function is not a function of a single structure. It results from the interplay of diverse cortical and subcortical structures, i.e., the prefrontal cortex (PFC), basal ganglia, and the cerebellum [40,41]. The various executive functions include reasoning, working memory, thinking, concept formation, inhibition, attention, abstraction, and modulation of social behavior [42]. Executive functions consist of high-level cognitive functions that are involved in the control and direction of lower-level functions [43]. Executive dysfunction is the most commonly encountered cognitive sequel in most of the acquired brain-damaged individuals. It is, therefore, imperative to understand the theoretical aspects of executive functions, the subcomponents of executive functions, and the neural circuitry that mediates these functions in order to improve these functions.

## Theories of Executive Functions

Executive functions are largely mediated by the PFC. Several influential theories have examined the function of the PFC. The supervisory attentional system (SAS) [44] posits that the frontal lobe is crucially involved in allocating attentional resources for processing information [5]. The model comprises four levels of increasing organization. The first level consists of cognitive or action units, which are the basic abilities such as reading a word or reaching for an object. The second level consists of schemas, or the thought representation. The third level is the process known as contention scheduling, which is the basic interface between incoming stimulus inputs, including thoughts, and the schemas. The cognitive system that effects the conscious deliberation is the supervisory attention system (SAS) which is the fourth level of processing. This SAS is thought to play an important role in eight different processes including working memory, monitoring and rejection of schema generation, adaptation of processing mode, goal setting, delayed intention marker realization, and episodic memory. However, the theory does not explain how the SAS operates, but only suggests that the SAS mediates novel activities such as planning of actions requiring conscious deliberation that are not available to the contention scheduling [45].

It is hypothesized [46] that the entire PFC is dedicated to memory, planning, or execution of actions. The orbital and the medial PFC, through its connections to the brain stem and limbic formation, plays a major role in emotional behavior and control of basic drives. The executive functions are carried out by the neural networks of the dorsolateral prefrontal cortex (DLPFC), subcortical structures, and association cortex. The main function of the lateral PFC is the temporal integration of information for attainment of prospective behavioral goals. This is complemented by working memory and preparatory set and is considered to be a temporally symmetric function, working together toward the goals in every sphere of action. The role of the DLPFC is hypothesized to be mediation of contingencies across time between event representation and the executive memory network in close interaction with the posterior cortex. The PFC integrates the cognitive representations of perception and action as required by goals of behavior.

An integrative theory of the PFC has been proposed [47] which attempts to explain how integration occurs in the PFC. The contention is that the PFC is not critical for performing simple, automatic behavior such as automatic orientation to sound or movement. Rather, the PFC serves a specific function in cognitive control and actively maintains patterns of activity that represent goals and the means to achieve them. This is done by directing the attentional resources towards the target stimuli, thus affecting the processing of the visual and the sensory modalities as well as systems responsible for response execution, memory retrieval, and emotional evaluation. The aggregate effect of the attentional bias is to guide the flow of neural activity along the pathways that establish the proper mapping between inputs, internal states, and outputs needed to perform a given task. This is essential when the stimulus is ambiguous, presumably activating more than one input representation. This may result in the possibility of multiple competing responses and strong alternatives. The constellation of the PFC resolves this competition, guides activity along appropriate pathways, and establishes the mapping needs to perform the task.

Given the important and crucial roles played by the DLPFC in particular and the PFC in general, one can assume that these areas are responsible for the smooth functioning of the executive system in everyday functioning. Lesion studies have shown that disruption of cognitive processes follow disruption of these specific areas or networks. Drawing heavily on this understanding, the clinical neuropsychological model helps to understand the brain–behavior relationship. It hypothesizes that a particular region of the brain is relevant to a particular function; damage to this distinct area would impair that function [48]. Neuropsychological test performance on large number of patients with focal lesions in different regions in the frontal lobe indicated that several regions of the frontal lobe are involved in a particular cognitive process. Conversely, a particular frontal region is involved in diverse cognitive processes. Lesion in the left dorsolateral prefrontal areas showed impairment in verbal processing, initiation, and switching; lesions in the right DLPFC caused impaired switching, sustaining, monitoring, and inhibition; inferior medial areas affect maintenance of information, inhibition, and explicit memory; superior medial regions in the PFC affect initiation, switching, and maintenance of information [48]. This suggests that the bilateral dorsolateral and inferior and superior medial regions are recruited in a single cognitive process and, conversely, a single frontal region has a role in computation of multiple cognitive processes. This is accomplished through complex interaction of neural circuitry.

## Neural Circuitry Mediating Executive Functions

The PFC is not homogenous and is thought to mediate different functions together with the subcortical nuclei such as basal ganglia and thalamus circuitry [40,49]. These include executive functions such as attention, response inhibition, mental flexibility, planning and organization, decision making, and emotional regulation. It also has a regulatory influence on the perceptual and sensory information received from the posterior regions [50]. The PFC, therefore, is considered to be a confluence of neural networks originating from the posterior regions [51] in view of the bidirectional connection of multiple areas of the brain.

Researchers have proposed five fronto-subcortical circuits; three of these circuits have been proposed to play a crucial role in regulating behavior and in mediating various functions. Executive functions are supported by the dorsolateral prefrontal circuits [40]. The orbitofrontal circuits mediate mood regulation, response inhibition, and socially appropriate behavior. The third circuit, involving the anterior cingulated, mediates the drive state, error monitoring, and response conflict resolution. Damage to this circuit leads to apathy, akinetic mutism, and reduced verbal output [40]. Damage to the right orbitofrontal area and its circuitry results in personality change. Disruption of any of these circuits results in corresponding cognitive deficits. Therefore, training the core components of the executive functions would not only improve the trained cognition but also the secondary cognitive functions such as memory and emotional regulation. It can be argued that training the executive functions could possibly enhance the overall functioning of frontal circuitry and its cortical and subcortical connection. Conversely, developing tasks that are mediated by the cortical and subcortical circuitry should enhance the executive functions in general and therefore enhance overall functioning and result in generalization to other cognitive processes such as memory as well as everyday functioning. Neuropsychological rehabilitation programs have been developed to stimulate the fronto-subcortical circuitry, using paper-and-pencil tasks to improve attention, response inhibition, temporal and spatial encoding, and divided attention tasks.

Kumar et al. (unpublished thesis) proposed a model to explain neuropsychological rehabilitation in traumatic brain-injury patients using a combination of information-processing theory and a neural circuitry and neuropsychological approach. This model draws its theoretical framework from the effortful and automatic processing models proposed by Schneider and Shiffrin [52] and Hasher and Zacks [53], as well as the more recent understanding of the neural circuitry that meditates cognitive functions.

The limited capacity theory describes two kinds of information processing: controlled or effortful processing and automatic processing [52,53]. Controlled or effortful processing places demands on the limited capacity or the attentional resources. Controlled processes include rehearsal, imagery, organization, mnemonics, sustained and focused attention, and processing of physical attributes of the environment [53,54]. Automatic processing places less demand on the attentional resources and has direct access to long-term memory. Thus, the components of memory such as temporal, spatial, and frequency information are encoded automatically. The temporal, spatial, and frequency aspects of information aid in the recall of events in memory [53]. There appears to be some overlap between executive functions and the controlled processes as both consist of subcomponents of goal-directed activities such as planning, organization, contextual memory, inhibition and fluency, self-regulation of affect, motivation, arousal, internalization of speech, and reconstitution of behavior through analysis and synthesis [55–58]. Neuropsychological and functional neuroimaging studies suggest that these cognitive process are mediated by the PFC [56,57] and its cortico-cortical connection from the posterior regions [51]. From the controlled and automatic process theory [52], constant practice of controlled processes allows the effortful process to become automatic and effortless [52,53]. From the contemporary neuropsychology perspective, these executive functions are mediated by the fronto-subcortical circuits [40,41]. Combining the two perspectives (Figure 6.1), it can be hypothesized that with constant practice of the executive functions, they can be made automatic and also possibly improve the functioning of the circuits that mediate these functions. Based on this rationale, a comprehensive neuropsychological rehabilitation program addressing various cognitive domains such as attention, executive functions, and memory is developed primarily for patients with traumatic brain injury, and subsequently extended to ameliorate cognitive deficits associated with other neurological conditions such as stroke and infectious diseases. It has been a challenge to develop cognitive retraining programs for Indian

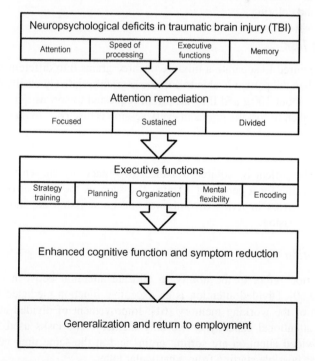

**Figure 6.1** Diagrammatic representation of the proposed model of rehabilitation.

populations from different socioeconomic strata and different levels of education. Developing rehabilitation programs for illiterate patients has been an especially unique experience. Efforts have been made to develop neuropsychological rehabilitation programs to suit patients from urban and rural backgrounds and different levels of education. The rehabilitation tasks have been developed using materials that are easily available to individuals from both urban and rural India. The hospital-based program requires the patients to come for rehabilitation on a daily basis for about 45 min to an hour. For the home-based program, the primary caregiver of the patient is included in the initial treatment program and subsequently trained to provide rehabilitation to the patient. Weekly or fortnightly contact with the patient and the caregiver is made to ensure adherence to the rehabilitation program. All the cognitive domains are addressed in the rehabilitation. Some of the rehabilitation tasks developed for patients with acquired brain damage are briefly described in the following section.

## Attention Training

Focused attention is defined as selectively reacting to stimuli in the presence of irrelevant stimuli having distracting potential. These irrelevant stimuli may be similar to the target stimuli [58]. Sustained attention refers to the ability to selectively attend to task-relevant information over a prolonged period of time. The task used for the improvement of sustained, focused, and divided attention include grain sorting, letter cancellation, and coloring.

### Grain Sorting Task

Patients are required to separate a mixture of three grains into different piles as fast as possible; when the patient is able to sort these grains relatively easily, the quantity is increased to about 100 g and they are again requested to sort as quickly as possible. The time taken to sort the grains in every session is disclosed to them.

### Letter Cancellation

On this task, the patient is required to cancel two randomly chosen vowels from a page of a magazine for a period of 15 min. The score is the number of letters cancelled, and the errors in terms of omission and commission are indicated to the patient in every session.

### Divided Attention

Divided attention refers to the ability to allocate attention between two concurrent tasks [59,60]. Divided attention is an executive function mediated by the central executive of the working memory [61]. Improvement of divided attention can improve the attentional capacity or working memory. The tasks used for training patients in divided attention are sorting grains and at the same time generating as many words as possible starting from a particular letter.

## Temporal Encoding

This task is aimed at making encoding of words automatic and effortless. In this task, the patient is presented with a list of words divided into three segments. The list is presented verbally at the rate of 2 s per word. After the list is read out, the patient is required to recall only the first two words. The same list is presented again and the patient is told to recall the last set of two words. The same procedure is followed for the middle two words. The patient is taught mnemonic strategies such as semantic elaboration, i.e., organizing the words into a meaningful sentence, and rehearsal for each segment of the list. On applying the strategies to all the segments of the list, the patient is asked to recall all the words. The strategies learned in the first list are applied to a new list of words. The scaffolding rendered to the patient is reduced as the patient gains mastery in the use of these strategies.

## Spatial Encoding

This task is aimed at making spatial encoding automatic. The patient is presented with six objects on a table for a duration of 15 s. After the exposure time, the objects are covered with a flat board, and the patient is asked to name and locate each object under the board. When patients are able to name and locate all the six objects under the board, the number of objects is increased gradually from 6 to 8, 10, 12, and 15.

## Self-Regulation Task

The coloring task is used as a task for self-regulation. An outline drawing of a design is presented to the patient. The patient is required to color it with colored pencil. The patient is required to maintain constant pressure of the pencil on the paper, make strokes as even as possible, and restrict the coloring to its respective boundaries. Initially, the patient is given simple drawings; when the patient shows improvement on the task, the complexity of the drawing is increased. Figure 6.2 describes the model to explain neuropsychological rehabilitation at different levels. Figure 6.3 depicts the neuropsychological rehabilitation tasks.

At the first level, attentional deficits are ameliorated by tasks such as letter cancellation, grain sorting, and coloring for a prolonged period of time. When the patient develops the ability to sustain attention on a particular task for a prolonged period of time, he/she also develops the ability to suppress and inhibit irrelevant or distracting stimuli by focusing on a particular target stimulus. For adequate inhibition, the patient should have adequate sustained attention. Ameliorating attention deficits through constant practice in daily sessions might bring about an optimal level of functioning in these cognitions [56,62,63]. Executive functions depend on effective response inhibition of irrelevant information. Therefore, it can be argued that the ability to sustain attention and inhibit irrelevant information results in adequate performance of executive function [56].

At the second level, with improvement in attention and ability to participate in a task adequately, encoding of contextual information such as temporal, spatial, and frequency encoding strategies are taught. In these tasks, especially the temporal

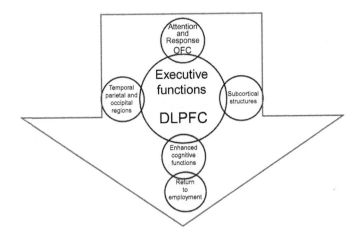

**Figure 6.2** Interaction between the functions addressed in the rehabilitation programme and the corresponding brain regions.

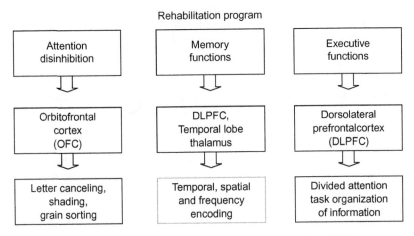

**Figure 6.3** Diagrammatic representation of the tasks addressed by the rehabilitation programme and the mediating anatomical regions.

encoding, executive functions like planning and organization of the word that has to be learned from the word list are trained. The patients are taught to develop and use their own strategies, such as associating the given set of words, semantic elaboration, and visualization. All the strategies used in encoding and retrieval, such as checking and monitoring, are part of the executive functions [63,64].

Temporal encoding also requires increasing loads of working memory for adequate performance, particularly when the number of words to learn and recall increases. On the first level of temporal encoding, the patient is presented with six words divided into three segments. The patient is required to hold in mind (online) the words learned in the first segment while manipulating the words in the second segment. On the third segment, the patient has to hold information learned in the first and the second segment as well. In spatial encoding, the patient has to remember the location of the object exposed and also name the object that was kept covered after exposure. On this level, additional tasks of executive functions such as design fluency and verbal fluency are trained.

When some patients do not improve despite practice at his level, then divided attention tasks requiring the patient to sort grain while simultaneously generating as many words as possible are continued, as in verbal/phonemic fluency.

At the third level, the level of difficulty is increased, including length of the word list for temporal encoding and making the words more abstract and thus more difficult to associate. Associating the abstract words requires greater levels of organization, planning, and working memory as they have to hold the segments in mind while working on the second or third set of words. Increased difficulty levels place greater demands on the central executive function [61]. The constant practice with increasing levels of difficulty results in enhanced performance, which may in turn augment the functioning of the neural circuitry recruited for these functions.

## Neuropsychological Rehabilitation Based on Neural Circuitry: Case Studies

The neuropsychological rehabilitation program based on the aforementioned model (Figure 6.1) has been applied to three different neurological conditions in the following section.

---

**Case 1**

Miss JM, a 27-year-old married female with no contributory past, family, or personal history, premorbidly well adjusted, working as a nurse, developed fever with myalgia and sore throat, a few days following which she was observed to exhibit odd behaviors. She became restless and irritable. MRI revealed bilateral medial temporal hyperintense signals, and EEG showed diffuse background slowing. Her sensorium improved and she became restless. She developed olfactory and hallucinatory behavior. She was referred to psychiatry for behavior problems. While she was under psychiatric treatment, she continued to be markedly agitated, experienced hallucination in multiple modalities, and had prominent affective lability. She was reported to be elated, frequently singing and dancing, and showed disinhibited, irritable, and violent behavior. She was referred for neuropsychological assessment and rehabilitation for memory problems.

She was not amenable to assessment. Hence, cognitive retraining was started based on clinical observations and interview. The aim was to enhance focused and sustained attention. She was given grain sorting and letter cancellation for focused and sustained attention. A shading task was used to enhance emotional regulation and response inhibition. The grain sorting comprised of three small grains mixed together. The patient had to sort the grains into three piles everyday as quickly as possible. Feedback about the performance and the time was given to the patient after every session. The letter-cancellation task required the patient to cancel two target letters, usually vowels from the running text on a given page in a magazine for a period of 15 min. The target letters were changed everyday. Following six sessions, the patient was amenable to a formal neuropsychological assessment. The assessment revealed severe memory deficits, with complete inability to recall any fact after a delay of 20 min in both verbal and visual memory tests (Figure 6.4). In addition to the attention and self-regulation tasks, memory encoding and retrieval tasks were administered. The memory tasks were temporal, spatial, and frequency encoding. The temporal encoding consisted of six words of four lists for the first 2 weeks. She was able to recall about three words but had difficulty recalling after 1-min delay. In the third week, she could recall all the six words, and the level of difficulty was increased to nine words. She made substantial gains on temporal encoding. She was discharged from the hospital but continued with a home-based cognitive training program for the next 6 months with monthly contact with the therapist during which the task difficulty was increased to 12 words. On reassessment, she showed significant improvement in cognitive functions and maintained the improvement at the 1-year follow-up.

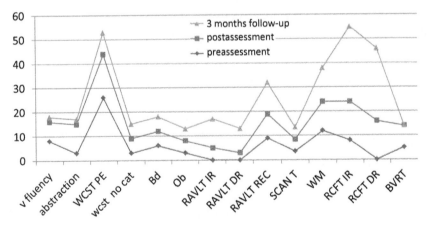

**Figure 6.4 Graph showing the scores of JM across the two assessments.** v fluency, verbal fluency; WCST PE, persistent errors on Wisconsin Card Sorting Test; wcst no cat, number of categories on Wisconsin Card Sorting test; Bd, block design test; Ob, object assembly test; RAVTL IR, immediate recall on Ray Auditory Verbal Learning Test; RAVLT Dr, delayed recall on Ray Auditory Verbal Learning Test; RAVLT REC, number of words correctly recognized on Ray Auditory Verbal Learning Test; SCAN T, time taken on trial making test; WM, working memory; RCFT IR, immediate recall on Rey Ostriech Complex Figure Test; RCFT Dr, delayed recall on Rey Ostriech Complex Figure Test; BVRT, Benton Visual Retention Test.

## Case 2

Mr. G, a 27-year-old unmarried male, a software engineer by profession, presented with a history of road traffic accident (RTA). Premorbidly he was well adjusted, with a good academic record, presented with history of left Arteriovenous malformation (AVM). His neuroimaging revealed a left frontoparietal hemorrhage. He presented with complaints of severe expressive speech difficulty and forgetting. There was a history of personality change in the form of increased irritability, and he would get frustrated easily.

A comprehensive neuropsychological assessment was attempted (Figure 6.5). His speech was not fluent and he had word-finding difficulty. His initial neuropsychological assessment revealed severely impaired working memory, phonemic fluency, and word-finding difficulty, with deficits in verbal learning and memory (RAVLT). His performance on these tests fell below the 5th percentile. He underwent a total of 60 sessions of neuropsychological rehabilitation. The program consisted of letter cancellation and shading for attention, temporal encoding for working memory, learning, and memory, as well as he was taught strategies for organization and association of words into meaningful sentences and visualization. The length of the word list was increased from 6 to 9 words,

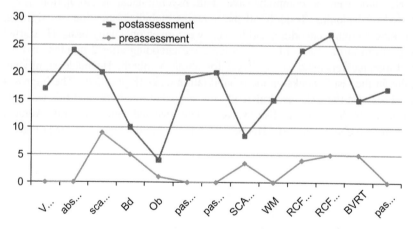

**Figure 6.5 Graph showing the scores of Mr. G across three assessments.** v fluency, verbal fluency; WCST PE, persistent errors on Wisconsin Card Sorting Tests; wcst no cat, number of categories on Wisconsin Card Sorting test Category; Bd, block design test; Ob, object assembly test; RAVTL IR, immediate recall on Ray Auditory Verbal Learning Test; RAVLT Dr, delayed recall on Ray Auditory Verbal Learning Test; RAVLT REC, number of words correctly recognized on Ray Auditory Verbal Learning Test; SCAN T, time taken on trial making test; WM, working memory; RCFT IR, immediate recall on Rey Ostriech Complex Figure Test; RCFT Dr, delayed recall on Rey Ostriech Complex Figure Test; BVRT, Benton Visual Retention Test.

12, and 15 words over a period of 60 sessions. Additional phonemic fluency tasks were given. The task required him to generate as many words as possible in 3 min. His postassessment revealed significant improvement on all the executive functions and the visual memory test (RCFT). However, he was able to learn only 9 out of 15 words on fifth trial of the RAVLT, and on the delayed recall after 20 min, he was able to recall all the 9 words.

### Case 3

Mr. S, a 39-year-old male, educated up to B.Tech., a software engineer by profession, right-handed individual, presented with a history of RTA in 2007, sustained head injury. He was reportedly under the influence of alcohol. He was presented with a history of loss of consciousness for one month and ENT bleeding. CT scan revealed acute subdural hematoma involving left fronto-temporo-parietal regions. With evidence of left temporal contusion, an emergency craniotomy was done. He was presented to the Neuropsychology Unit, NIMHANS, with right-side weakness, slurring of speech, word-finding difficulty, anterior grade and retrograde amnesia, delusion of persecution, and increased irritability with the slightest provocation. His initial neuropsychological assessment revealed severe deficits on all the tests, with scores of zero. He could get all the block designs correctly.

He underwent a comprehensive neuropsychological rehabilitation for a period of 4 months. Tasks in all the domains including attention, set shifting, working memory, encoding, and fluency were given on a daily basis. He started to perform at the 12-word level on temporal encoding after 2 months, and his performance remained at this level for about a month. He made significant gains in the last 2 weeks on the rehabilitation tasks (Figure 6.6). The improvement seen on the tasks generalized to his everyday functions, and this was corroborated by his parents. His postassessment revealed significant improvement on neuropsychological tests. His performance fell in the above-average range.

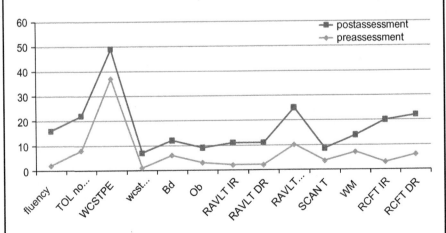

**Figure 6.6** Graph showing the scores of Mr. S across two assessments.

# Conclusion

- Neuropsychological rehabilitation as an intervention method to improve cognitive functions following neurological conditions, particularly for traumatic brain injury, is well established.
- Despite enhanced understanding of the mechanism of the recovery, there is no clear consensus as to how to rehabilitate cognitive sequelae of neurological conditions.
- With advances in neuroscience and use of neuroimaging techniques, there are strong indications that a circuit-based approach may be a useful method to rehabilitating cognitive deficits.
- Training of the dysfunctional circuits by means of cognitive exercises and strategy training might rewire and accommodate improvement in cognitive functions in a way that is similar to healthy normals.
- Preliminary studies at the NIMHANS has attempted to use a circuitry-based rehabilitation program in several neurological conditions such as stroke, traumatic brain injury, and infectious diseases, with promising results.
- However, there is a great need for more studies replicating and improving this method of neuropsychological rehabilitation.

# References

[1] Rizzo, M., & Tranel, D. (1996). *Head injury and post concussive syndrome*. New York: Churchill Livingstone.

[2] Anderson, T., Heitger, M., & Macleod, A. D. (2006). Concussion and mild head injury. *Practical Neurology, 6*, 342–357.

[3] Levin, H. S., Gary, E. H., Howard, M., Eisenberg, H. M., Ruff, R. M., Barth, J. T., et al. (1990). Neurobehavioural outcome 1 year after severe head injury. *Journal of Neurosurgery, 73*, 699–709.

[4] Van der Sluis, C. K., Eisma, W. H., Groothoff, J. W., & ten Duis, H. J. (1998). Long-term physical, psychological and social consequences of severe injuries. *Injury, 29*(4), 281–285.

[5] Ciceron, K. D., Mott, T., Azulay, J., Sharlow-galella, M. A., Ellimo, W., Paradise, S., et al. (2008). Randomizedd control trail of holistic neuriologic rehabilitation after traumatic brain injury. *Archives of Physical Medicine and Rehabilitation, 89*(December), 2239–22492.

[6] Rose, F. C., & Symonds, C. P. (1960). Persistent memory deficits following encephalitis. *Brain, 83*, 195–212. 13.

[7] Kapur, N., Barker, S., & Burrows, E. H. (1994). Herpes simplex encephalitis: Long term magnetic resonance imaging and neuropsychological profile. *JNNP, 57*, 1334–1342.

[8] Hierons, R., Janota, I., & Corsellis, J. A. (1978). The late effects of necrotizing encephalitis of the temporal lobes and limbic areas; a clinic-pathological study of 10 cases. *Psychological Medicine, 8*(21–24), 11.

[9] Hokkanen, L., Poutiainen, E., Valanne, L., Solonen, O., Iivanainen, M., & Launes, J. (1996). Cognitive impairment after acute encephalitis: Comparison of herpes simplex with other aetiologies. *Journal of Neurology, Neurosurgery and Psychiatry, 61*, 478–484.

[10] Barba, R., Martinez-Espinosa, T., Rodriguez-Garcia, E., Pondal, M., Vivancos, J., & Del Ser, T. (2000). Postdtroke dementia: Clinical features and risk factors. *Stroke, 31*, 1494–1501.

[11] Pohjasvaara, T., Erkinjuntti, T., Vataja, R., & Kaste, M. (1997). Dementia three months after stroke: Baseline frequency and effet of different definition of dementia in Helsinki stroke aging memory study (SAM) cohort. *Stroke, 28,* 785–792.

[12] Tatemichi, T. K., Desmond, D. W., Stern, T., Sano, M., Mayeur, R., & Andrews, H. (1992). Prevalence of dementia after stroke depends on diagnostic criteria. *Neurology, 42,* 413.

[13] Hachinski, V., Iadecola, C., Petersen, R., Breteler, M. M., Nyenhuis, D. L., Black, S., et al. (2006). National institute of neurological disorders and stroke- Canadian stroke network vascular impairment harmonization standards. *Stroke, 37,* 2220–2241.

[14] Sohlberg, M. M., & Mateer, C. A. (1987). Effectiveness of an attentional training program. *Journal of Clinical Experimental Neuropsychology, 9,* 117–130.

[15] Ponsford, J. L., & Kinsella, G. (1988). Evaluiation of a remedial program for attentional deficits following closed head injury. *Journal Clinical and Experimental Neuropsychobiology, 10,* 51–52.

[16] Ben-Yishay, Y., Piasetsky, E., & Rattock, J. (1987). A systematic method for ameliorating disorders in basic attention. In M. Meier, A. C. Benton, & L. Diller. (Eds.), *Neuropsychological rehabilitation.* New York: Churchill Livingstone.

[17] Sivak, M., Hill, C. S., & Olson, P. L. (1984). Computerized video tasks as training techniques for driving-related perceptual deficits of persons with brain damage: A pilot evaluation. *International Journal of Rehabilitation, 7,* 389–398.

[18] Wood, R., & Fussey, I. (1987). Computer based retraining; a controlled study. *International Disability Studies, 9,* 149–153.

[19] Malec, J., Jones, R., Rao, N., & Strubbs, K. (1984). Video game, practice effect on sustained attention in patients with cranio cerebral trauma. *Cognitive Rehabilitation, 2,* 18–23.

[20] Patten, B. M. (1972). The ancient art of memory: Usefulness and treatment. *Archives of Neurology, 26,* 28–31.

[21] Levinsohn, P. M., Danaher, B. G., & Kikel, S. (1977). Visual imagery as a mnemonic aid for brain injured persons. *Journal of Consulting and Clinical Psychology, 45,* 717–723.

[22] Glasgow, R. E., Zeiss, R. A., Barrera, M., & Lewinsohn, P. M. (1977). Case studies on remediating memory deficits in brain damaged individuals. *Journal of Clinical Psychology, 33*(4), 1049–1054.

[23] Crovitz, H. F., Harvey, M. T., & Horn, R. W. (1979). Problems in the acquisition of imagery mnemonics: Three brain damaged cases. *Cortex, 15,* 225–234.

[24] Graffman, J., & Mathew, C. (1978). Assessment and remediation of memory deficits in brain –injured patients. In M. Gruneberg, P. Mocris, & R. Sykes. (Eds.), *Practicle aspects of memory* (pp. 720–728). London: Academic Press.

[25] Glisky, E. L., Schater, D. L., & Tulving, E. (1986). Learning and retention of computer related vocabulary in memory impaired patients. Method of vanishing cues. *Journal of Clinical Experimental Neuropsychology, 8,* 292–312.

[26] Sholberg, M. M., & Mateer, C. A. (1989). *Introduction to cognitive rehabilitation. Theory and practice.* New York: Guilford Press.

[27] Cicerone, K. D., & Wood, J. C. (1987). Planning disorder after head injury: A case study. *Archives of Physical and Medical Rehabilitation, 68,* 111–115.

[28] Von Cramon, D., Von Cramon, G., & Mai, N. (1991). Problem solving deficits in brain injured patients: A therapeutic approach. *Neuropsychological Rehabilitation, 1*(1), 45–64.

[29] Batchelor, J., Shores, E., Marrosszeky, J., Sandman, J., & Lovarini, M. (1988). Cognitive rehabilitation of severely head-injured patients using computer-assisted and noncomputerized treatment techniques. *Journal of Head Trauma Rehabilitation, 3,* 78–83.

[30] Chen, S. G. A., Glueckauf, R. L., & Bracy, O. L. (1997). The effectiveness of computer-assisted cognitive rehabilitation for persons with traumatic brain injury. *Brain Injury, 2,* 197–209.

[31] Nag-Arulmani, S., & Rao, S. L. (1999). Remediation of attention deficits in head injury. *Neurology India, 47,* 32–39.

[32] Misra, S., & Rao, S. L. (1994). Divided attention in head injury. *NIMHANS Journal, 12*(2), 157–162.

[33] Kumar, K. J. Rao, S. L., & Chandramouli, B. A. (2005). Innovative methods of rehabilitation in head injury. Paper presented in World Congress in Brain Injury, Melbourne, Australia.

[34] Kumar, K. J.. (2007). Neuropsychological rehabilitation: A functional neural network approach. Continuing Neuropsychological Education (CEN), NIMHANS, Bangalore, India.

[35] Rao, S. L., Gangadhar, B. N., & Hegde, A. S. (1986). Information processing deficits as diagnostic tools in post concussion syndrome. *Neurology India, 34,* 271–274.

[36] Shylaja, K., & Mukundan, C. R. (2003). Computer aided cognitive retraining for head injured patients. Unpublished M. Phil. dissertation submitted to Department of Mental Health and Social Psychology. NIMHANS, Bangalore, Karnataka, India.

[37] Robertson, I. H., & Murre, J. M. J. (1999). Rehabilitation of brain damage: Brain plasticity and principles of guided recovery. *Psychological Bulletin, 125*(5), 544–575.

[38] Mateer, C. A., & Mapou, R. L. (1996). Understanding, evaluating and managing attention disorders following traumatic brain injury. *Journal of Head Trauma Rehabilitation, 11,* 1–16.

[39] Lezak, M. D. (1995). *Neuropsychological assessment* (3rd ed.). New York: Oxford University Press.

[40] Cummings, J. L. (1993). Frontal subcortical circuits and human behaviour. *Archives of Neurology, 50,* 873–880.

[41] Tekin, S., & Cummings, J. L. (2002). Frronto-subcortical neuronal circuits and clinical neuropsychiatry: An update. *Journal of Psychosomatic Research, 53,* 647–654.

[42] Grafman, J. (2002). The structured event complex and the human prefrontal complex. In D. T. Stuss, & R. T. Knight (Eds.), *Principles of frontal lobe function.* New York: Oxford University Press.

[43] Stuss, D. T., & Levine, B. (2002). Adult clinical neuropsychological: Lessons from studies of the frontal lobes. *Annual Review of Psychology.*

[44] Shallice, T. (1998). *From neuropsychology to mental structure.* Cambridge: Cambridge University Press.

[45] Shallice, T. (2002). Fractionating of the supervisory system. In D. T. Stuss & R. T. Knight (Eds.), *Principles of frontal lobe function.* New York: Oxford University Press.

[46] Fuster, J. M. (2001). The prefrontal cortex-an update: Time is of the essence. *Neuron, 30,* 319–333.

[47] Miller, E. K., & Cohen, J. D. (2001). An integrative theory of prefrontal cortex function. *Annual Review of Neuroscience, 24,* 167–202.

[48] Stuss, D. T., Alexander, M. P., Floden, D., Binns, M. A., Levine, B., McIntosh, A. R., et al. (2002). Fractionation and localization of distinct frontal lobe processes: Evidence from focal lesions in humans. In D. T. Stuss & R. T. Knight (Eds.), *Principles of frontal lobe function.* New York: Oxford University Press.

[49] Alexander, G. E., Delaneyy, M. R., & Strick, P. L. (1990). Parallel organisations of functionally segregated circuits linking basal cortex and cortex. *Annals Review Neuroscience, 9,* 357–358.

[50] D'Esposito, M., Aguirre, G. K., Zarahn, E., Ballard, D., Shin, R. K., & Lease, J. (1998). Functional MRI studies of spatial and non-spatial working memory. *Cognitive Brain Research, 7,* 1–13.

[51] Petride, M., & Pandya, D. (2002). In D. T. Stuss & R. T. Knight (Eds.), *Principles of frontal lobe function.* New York: Oxford University Press.

[52] Schneider, W., & Shiffrin, (1977), Controlled and automatic human information processing I. Detection, search, and attention. *Psychological Review, 84,* 1–60.

[53] Hasher, L., & Zacks, R. T. (1979). Automatic and effortful processes in memory. *Journal of Experimental Psychology, General, 108,* 356–388.

[54] Dark, J. D., Johnston, W. A., Worsley., M. M., & Farah, M. J. (1985). Levels of selection and capacity limits. *Journal of Experimental Psychology: General, 114*(4), 472–497.

[55] Pennington, B. F., & Ozonoff, S. (1996). Executive functions and developmental psychopathology. *Journal of Child Psychology and Psychiatry, 12*(1), 52–87.

[56] Barkley, R. A. (1997). Behavioral inhibition, sustained attention, and executive function: Constructing a unifying theory of ADHD. *Psychological Bulletin, 121*(1–2), 65–94.

[57] Duncan, J., & Owen, A. M. (2000). Common regions of the human frontal lobe recruited by diverse cognitive demands. *Trends in Neurosciences, 23,* 475–483.

[58] Van Zomeren, A. H., & Fasotti, L. (1992). Impairments of attention in brain damaged patients. In N. Von Steiinbuchel, D. Y. Von cramon, & E. Poppel (Eds.), *Neuropsychological rehabilitation.* Berlin/Heidelberg: Springer-Verlag.

[59] Friedman, A. B., & Polson, M. C. (1981). Hemisphere as independent resource system: Limited capacity processing abd cerebral specialization. *Journal of Experimental Psychology: Human Perception and Performance, 7,* 1031–1058.

[60] Friedman, A. B., Polson, M. C., Defoe, C. G., & Gaskill, S. J. (1982). Dividing attention with and between hemispheres: Testing a multiple resource approach to limited capacity information processing. *Journal of Experimental Psychology: Human Perception and Performance, 8,* 625–650.

[61] D'Esposito, M., Detre, J. A., Alsop, D. C., Shin, R. K., Atlas, S., & Grossman, M. (1995). The Neural basis of the central executive system of working memory. *Nature, 378,* 279–281.

[62] Starkstein, S. E., & Robinson, R. G. (1997). Mechanism of disinhibition after brain lesions. *Journal of Nervous and Mental Disease, 185*(2), 108–113.

[63] Fletcher, P. C., Shallice, T., & Dolan, R. J. (1998). The functional roles of prefrontal cortex in episodic memory. I. *Encoding Brain, 121,* 1239–1248.

[64] Buckner, R. C., Kelly, W. M., & Peterson, S. E. (1999). Frontal cortex contribution to human memory formation. *Nature Neuroscience, 2,* 4.

# 7 Cognitive Remediation of Neurocognitive Deficits in Schizophrenia

S. Hegde*, S.L. Rao*, A. Raguram†,
B.N. Gangadhar‡

*Cognitive Psychology Unit, Centre for Cognition and Human Excellence, National Institute of Mental Health and Neurosciences (NIMHANS), Bangalore, Karnataka, India, †Department of Clinical Psychology, National Institute of Mental Health and Neurosciences (NIMHANS), Bangalore, Karnataka, India, ‡Department of Psychiatry, National Institute of Mental Health and Neurosciences (NIMHANS), Bangalore, Karnataka, India

Schizophrenia is one of the most debilitating illnesses. The illness is characterized by a group of symptoms clustered as positive and negative symptoms. Positive symptoms include hallucinations, delusions, incoherent speech, and even catatonic behavior. Negative symptoms include apathy, paucity of speech, blunting or incongruity of emotional responses, social withdrawal, and decline in social performance. The diagnosis of schizophrenia is made when the symptoms are present for a period of over 1 month (ICD-10, World Health Organization) [1] to 6 months (DSM-IV, American Psychiatric Association) [2]. The incidence of schizophrenia is 7 per 1000. The illness is most often observed in the age group of 15–35 years (WHO, 2012) [110]. In India, the annual incidence is 0.35–0.38 per 1000 in urban population and 0.44 per 1000 in the rural population [3]. Prevalence studies have reported 2.3 per 1000 with a range of 1.1–14.2 across studies [4].[1] There is no difference between the prevalence of the illness among males versus females or between urban/rural and mixed areas [5]. According to the recent report, schizophrenia affects nearly 24 million people across the globe [110]. Although the incidence rate is low, the prevalence of schizophrenia is high due to chronicity of the illness. The direct and indirect cost for both the society at large and for the patient and the caregivers of the patients is a major concern with this illness. The fact that the illness is manifested in adolescence and early adulthood, affecting overall functioning, and the fact that nearly two-thirds of the patients continue to have persistent or fluctuating symptoms despite psychopharmacological

---

[1] The term "prevalence" refers to the estimated population of people living with schizophrenia at any given time. The term "incidence" refers to the annual diagnosis rate, or the number of new cases of schizophrenia diagnosed each year.

Neuropsychological Rehabilitation-Principles and Applications.
DOI: http://dx.doi.org/10.1016/B978-0-12-416046-0.00007-9

treatment are the two main reasons why the illness causes such a burden. For instance, the total annual cost for the care of 50 outpatients in India was assessed at US$274. Indirect costs were assessed higher than the direct costs. The financial burden was borne by the family, and the increase in cost related positively with the chronicity of the illness with higher disability [6]. The treatment of this disabling illness has been a major challenge to mental health professionals and clinicians around the globe.

During the early 1950s, the focus of treatment for schizophrenia was chiefly on positive symptoms such as hallucinations and delusions using antipsychotics. The focus shifted toward treatment of negative symptoms such as anhedonia, avolition, and apathy in the 1980s, as negative symptoms were observed to be closely associated with functional recovery. Although positive symptoms, and to a certain extent negative symptoms, were treated via the psychopharmacological treatment, functional recovery of patients continued to pose a challenge to clinicians. Reduction of positive or negative symptoms did not lead to improvement in functional recovery or overall functioning such as everyday living skills or independence in living in the social and work domains [7]. A decade later, in the 1990s, the focus shifted to the role of neurocognitive deficits in schizophrenia. Neurocognitive deficits present in patients with schizophrenia were observed to be intimately related to the functional outcome of the illness [8,9]. Neurocognitive deficits were considered the core and enduring feature of the illness.

Presence of neurocognitive deficits in schizophrenia is not a recent observation. In the initial case accounts made by Kraepelin and Bleuler, deficits in attention, higher mental functions, and volition were considered important features of the illness. Schizophrenia was earlier known as *dementia precoce*, a term coined by Morel to describe the syndrome that included a progressive decline in function. The term was later translated by Kraepelin as *dementia precox*. He described the early or premature deterioration of functioning in this psychiatric illness. Bleuler, a Swiss psychiatrist, in 1911 coined the term "schizophrenia" and considered cognitive impairment a core feature of the illness. The emphasis on the presence of cognitive deficits was lost amid the primary focus on treating positive and negative symptoms using pharmacological means. With poor functional recovery of the illness and thereby increased overall cost of illness, cognitive deficits were reconsidered. Research studies in this area over the past three decades have reinstated neurocognitive deficits as an important illness feature, similar to positive and negative symptoms [10]. The current understanding is that schizophrenia is a disorder of the brain and that the underlying brain dysfunction is manifested as cognitive dysfunction [11]. A major shift has occurred from the initial understanding of schizophrenia as a neurodevelopmental, neurodegenerative disorder to what is known today as a neurocognitive disorder [12].

# Neurocognitive Deficits in Schizophrenia

Neurocognitive functions form the edifice for all our functioning and survival. Cognition is the term that encompasses all the functions required to understand and respond to the environment, thereby ensuring our survival. It, therefore, includes abilities that help us grasp the information from the environment, to attend to certain aspects of the environment in a focused way, to comprehend and make meaning of the information received via language or nonverbal modes, to be able to solve problems, to plan future actions, to evaluate our own thought processes, and so forth. Neurocognitive functions include processes like attention, information processing, comprehension, working memory, planning, concept formation, learning, memory, and insight.

Studies have demonstrated neurocognitive deficits in schizophrenia, using standardized neuropsychological assessment tools and methods. Patients with schizophrenia tend to perform poorer than do normal controls on a wide array of cognitive tasks [13–15]. The overall deficit is up to one standard deviation or more below the normal control population [16,17]. Deficits are present in sustained attention [18], working memory [19], auditory and visual information processing [20], verbal memory [21], impairment in executive functions [22], set shifting [23], planning [24], and insight into one's own clinical condition [25]. Deficits in attention and information processing are considered central to the disorder, and these contribute to deficits in working memory and executive functions [26]. Deficits are also observed in more complex measures of social cue recognition and "theory of mind" [27]. These cognitive deficits can be grouped into three major categories: (1) primary processes, including attention, information processing, and perception; (2) secondary processes, including executive functions and memory; and (3) metaprocesses, including insight [28, 111].

Much of the research over the last few decades has been directed toward understanding the nature of neurocognitive deficits in schizophrenia. Although the prevalence of schizophrenia is estimated to be lower in least developed countries compared to emerging and developed countries [5], and outcome has been reported to be poorer in developed countries compared to developing countries like India, the profile of cognitive deficits across countries with different economic status is reported to be similar [29]. There have been relatively few studies from India examining cognitive deficits in schizophrenia and also examining the relation between cognitive deficits and demographic variables [30–34]. In one study, 49 first-episode schizophrenia (FES) patients with less than 2 years of illness were assessed on a comprehensive battery of neuropsychological tests, the positive and negative syndrome scale [35] and the WHO Disability Assessment Schedule [36]. The cognitive deficit profile was drawn comparing the obtained score with Indian norms. A cognitive deficit quotient for each patient was calculated. Of the sample, 16.3% had less than 25% of cognitive deficits, 38.8% had 25–50% of cognitive deficits, 36.7% of them had 50–75% of cognitive deficits, and 8.2% had more than 75% cognitive deficits. More than 50% of the patients showed deficits in the domains of attention, executive functions, learning, and memory. Psychopathology significantly correlated with global functioning of these individuals. Negative symptoms significantly correlated with cognitive deficits of motor speed, attention, and executive functions [34]. In a study carried out on 100 chronic schizophrenia patients, subjects were assessed on a standard neuropsychological tests and were compared with a control group matched by age, gender, and education. The results showed neurocognitive deficits in the domains of attention, executive functions, and verbal learning and memory in the chronically ill schizophrenia patients [30]. Deficits in visual information processing assessed using simple reaction time, choice reaction time, and a forced span of apprehension test are reported in patients in remission [31]. Patients in the remission stage of the illness also have deficits in attention, executive functions, learning, and memory [37]. Neurocognitive deficits are present in the prodromal, psychotic, and chronic phases of schizophrenia. Deficit in cognitive performance is one of the manifestations of the neuropathology of the illness [38]. Impairment of neurocognitive functions as assessed on the standardized neuropsychological tests indicates a direct link to disturbed brain function [39]. Cognitive variables appear to be important endophenotypes for schizophrenia [40]. Structural and functional imaging studies have shown unequivocally that structural brain abnormalities exist in schizophrenia [41–43].

The main focus, however, is no longer whether there is any brain abnormality in schizophrenia, but understanding the nature of the neurocognitive deficits that are the manifestation of the underlying brain abnormalities and how these are related to the etiology, clinical features, and outcome of the illness. Cognitive deficits play a central role in deciding the course and outcome of this debilitating illness, mediated by impaired work performance, community functioning, social problem solving, and social skill acquisition [8,44–47]. A meta-analysis reported that cognitive deficits explained 20–60% of the variance in measured outcomes [9]. Cognitive functions also play an important role in the ability to benefit from other treatment modalities such as social skills training [48] or work rehabilitation [49]. Despite methodological variability across studies, there is consistency in reporting the presence of cognitive deficits in early phases of the illness. It is only in the recent past that concrete effort has been made to understand the functional implications of these deficits [8,50].

## Cognitive Remediation: A Treatment Method to Ameliorate Cognitive Deficits

Cognitive remediation seeks to ameliorate cognitive deficits. Cognitive remediation is a treatment strategy that involves psychological methods aiming at restoration of cognitive functions in brain-damaged patients. These are approaches to improve cognitive functioning that have been drawn from treatment of patients with traumatic brain injury or stroke. This method includes repeatedly practicing tasks—paper-and-pencil or computerized tasks that load on attention, memory, reasoning, or other specific cognitive functions [51,52]. Cognitive remediation targets to improve cognitive functions such as attention, speed of processing of information, and executive functions. It uses graded tasks to improve specific cognitive functions. The assumption is that improvements in basic functions generalize to the improvement of overall functioning [53]. The goal of cognitive remediation is, therefore, to produce both lasting improvement in the cognitive functions themselves and to generalize the improvement to reduce continuing weakness in other areas.

# Cognitive Remediation in Schizophrenia

The increasing awareness of the central role of cognitive deficits in schizophrenia has fostered considerable interest in the prospects for cognitive rehabilitation. Cognitive remediation for schizophrenia grew out of research documenting the success of such training in brain-injured patients and also out of research carried out in experimental psychopathology laboratories where researchers observed that manipulations of experimental stimuli (e.g., reduction in attentional demands and changes in stimulus characteristics) could produce improvements on laboratory tasks (for a review, refer to Ref. [54]). The initial studies to investigate the generalization of cognitive retraining to tasks other than specifically trained functions in patients with schizophrenia were carried out by Wagner (1968) [112] and Meichenbaum (1973) [113]. Almost a decade later, two studies rekindled interest in the application of cognitive retraining in schizophrenia. Goldberg et al. [55] reported that patients with schizophrenia were unable to benefit from explicit instructions and practice on the Wisconsin Card Sorting Test (WCST), the putative neuropsychological marker of prefrontal function. The results from the study [55] found poor levels of improvement. The authors concluded that a basic neurocognitive deficit owing to brain dysfunction made such rehabilitation impossible. Many studies following this showed the performance of schizophrenia patients on the WCST could be improved by training using different instruction conditions and reinforcement. A meta-analysis has reported efforts to improve WCST performance in the laboratory were successful, with a weighted mean effect size of 0.96 (Cohen's $d$) [56]. Several studies since then have been carried out to look at the effectiveness of cognitive rehabilitation in schizophrenia. In the past decade, studies on cognitive remediation in schizophrenia have multiplied and are still growing exponentially [57].

Cognitive remediation studies in schizophrenia have followed two approaches: laboratory and clinical (for a detailed review refer to Ref. [57]). The first approach includes studies carried out in laboratory settings with the aim of improving a single task or a component of tasks without integrating with a general rehabilitation program. Many of these studies have focused on improving cognitive functions on a neuropsychological test used to measure the same cognitive function. Examples are the following studies. Retraining was given on the WCST, incorporating strategic training and positive and monetary feedback [58,59]. However, the improvement was not sustained and failed to generalize to other problem-solving measures [55,60,61]. For a detailed review on this topic, refer to Kurtz et al. [56]. Cognitive training programs have been shown to improve the targeted function such as attention [62,63]; working memory [64] and emotion perception [65] have also been improved in schizophrenia patients through cognitive retraining. Cognitive retraining improves sustained attention and language processing [66], executive function [67], affect recognition, verbal memory [68,69], working memory [70,71], processing speed [68], and social problem solving [72]. The main challenge of this approach has been sustainability and generalizability of the improvement observed to overall functioning of the patient.

Significant impact on functional outcome and effective remediation of cognitive deficits has been increasingly cited as an essential component of comprehensive treatment. There is a need for integrated studies of cognitive retraining with other treatment programs, such as pharmacological management, psychoeducation, social skills training, work therapy, and family intervention. Improvement in overall functioning is perhaps achieved not just by cognitive retraining alone but also by targeting several other domains of dysfunctions observed in schizophrenia patients.

The second approach consists of comprehensive programs that include other training programs such as social skills training and work training along with cognitive remediation. This approach uses a number of different types of cognitive retraining programs, such as paper-and-pencil tasks, computer-based tasks, and group activities [73]. Integrated psychological therapy (IPT) [74], cognitive enhancement therapy (CET) [75], neurocognitive enhancement therapy [76], cognitive remediation therapy [77], and the neuropsychological educational approach to remediation [78] are some of the popular comprehensive programs.

Review studies of randomized clinical trials offer several important observations about cognitive remediation as a scientific endeavor. Meta-analysis of studies on cognitive remediation in schizophrenia [54] have found 17 randomized clinical trials in the literature and calculated weighted mean effect sizes (Cohen's $d$). The effect sizes were 0.32 for improvements in neuropsychological performance, 0.26 for reductions in symptom severity, and 0.51 for improvements in everyday function. However, only three studies have examined functional outcomes. Of these, only one study involving environmental manipulation found an effect size 0.58. The review studies reveal that very little evidence exists for cognitive remediation effects beyond such proximal outcomes as improvement on trained tasks or on closely related but untrained neuropsychological tests. McGurk et al. [79] conducted a meta-analysis of 26 randomized, controlled trials of cognitive remediation in schizophrenia, including 1151 patients. This study evaluated the effects of cognitive remediation for improving cognitive performance, symptoms, and psychosocial functioning in schizophrenia. Cognitive remediation was associated with significant improvements across all three outcomes, with a medium effect size for cognitive performance (0.41), a slightly lower effect size for psychosocial functioning (0.36), and a small effect size for symptoms (0.28) [79]. The effects of cognitive remediation on psychosocial functioning were significantly stronger in studies that provided adjunctive psychiatric rehabilitation than in studies that provided cognitive remediation alone. Cognitive remediation produced moderate improvements in cognitive performance and, when combined with psychiatric rehabilitation, also improved functional outcomes. Impact of cognitive remediation on functioning was moderated by provision of adjunctive psychiatric rehabilitation, cognitive training method, and patients' age. Improvements and generalization of the improvement to overall functioning have been the greatest challenge. Studies on the outcome of cognitive retraining indicate task-specific improvement but variable generalization to overall functioning [80].

As mentioned earlier in the text, the prevalence of schizophrenia does not differ widely across the globe. Theoretically, therefore, the treatment approaches too need not vary. However, in reality this is not the case. The difference in psychopharmacological treatment may be less compared to the difference in the method of other rehabilitation programs for schizophrenia. This is true of cognitive remediation programs as well. Until recently there were no systematically developed cognitive remediation programs suitable for patients in developing countries like India [33,81]. For instance, well-established programs such as IPT or CET pose practical challenges when implemented in a country like India. These training programs are group therapy programs varying from 9 months to 2 years in duration. Unlike patients in the Western countries, patients in a country like India generally do not receive any welfare benefits or financial support from insurance companies. More often than not it is the family that bears the entire treatment cost. In many cases, the patient is the breadwinner in family. Approximately 90% of patients with schizophrenia live with their families [82]. Family plays an important role in all stages of intervention. Often this kind of involvement is not merely because of close relationships but also due to lack of community-based or other treatment facilities. Family plays an important role in choice of drug, patient's compliance with drug, regular hospital visits, and it plays an important role in making decisions around the patient's life events such as work and marriage [83].

Family intervention was considered an important part of the intervention in this program as family environment is considered an important factor influencing the course and outcome of the illness. Family members do not just passively suffer the symptoms of the illness, but are often actively involved in coping with it [84]. Caregivers of the patients experience a period of disorganization and disruption as a consequence of the illness and disturbed interactions [85]. They experience upheavals in their personal lives and they experience burdens and changes in quality of life. Psychoeducation provides information regarding symptoms and behaviors associated with the illness and aids in better understanding how to deal with disturbing behaviors of the patient. Patients with schizophrenia and their families benefit from education and feedback regarding the illness, prognosis, and treatment. The addition of psychoeducation to the treatment program has shown significant reduction in relapse and readmission rates and improved family well-being [86,87]. Family interventions enhance understanding of the illness among the caregivers and foster supportive relationships in the family [88]. The anxiety, distress, and burden of the caregivers lessen and their acceptance of the patient's illness improves after family intervention [89].

Perhaps one of the reasons for poor generalization of improved cognitive functions following cognitive remediation may be the lack of a family environment to nurture and support the improvement. Improvement in cognitive function via cognitive remediation programs in schizophrenia is perhaps slow and gradual compared with conditions such as head injury. Family members may be unable to perceive the gradual and subtle improvements and hence fail to provide positive feedback to the patients. However, those families that recognize the improvements may develop excessively high expectations about the patients' level of clinical improvement and their general functioning. Either way, the consequences are likely to result in high-expressed emotions that could then have a deleterious impact on the gains acquired through the retraining program. A way out of this intractable situation would be family intervention. Thus, to optimize the clinical benefits for the patient, a combination of cognitive retraining and family intervention was considered since this approach would improve the cognitive functions of the schizophrenic patient and sustain the gains with a congenial family environment. The integrated psychological intervention (IPI) is a hospital-based 6-week paper-and-pencil-based cognitive remediation program, integrated with a biweekly family intervention program. This program has shown promising results in chronically ill schizophrenia patients [33].

## Cognitive Remediation Using the Integrated Psychological Intervention Program: A Case Illustration

In the 6-week-long, paper-and-pencil-based cognitive remediation programs, the tasks were arranged in increasing difficulty levels, and higher-level cognitive functions were targeted following remediation of basic functions. The functions of attention, fluency, information processing, working memory, and response inhibition were targeted in week 1. Tasks to improve the functions of visual immediate memory and spatial encoding were added in week 2. Finally, tasks to improve the functions of set shifting, planning, comprehension, and production of emotions were added in week 3. The cognitive retraining was carried out daily for 1½–2 h. Feedback on the performance of the retraining tasks was given at the end of each session. Details of the task and the schedule of the cognitive retraining program are presented in Table 7.1.

Family intervention was held biweekly. A total of 12 sessions were carried out with the primary caregivers of the patient. The intervention program was divided into four main phases. The first phase focused on assessment of the current functioning of the family. The second phase focused on providing the caregivers with basic knowledge regarding the illness as well as understanding of the role of cognitive deficits present in the patients and the role they have in the patient's overall functioning. Phase three focused on normalizing family routines, lowering of expressed emotions by the caregivers, and daily activity scheduling for the patient. Phase four focused on improving communication and problem-solving skills of the family members as well helping the caregiver find healthy support systems. The intervention also focused on clarifying any queries the caregivers had regarding the illness.

*Tools and measures used at preintervention, postintervention, and at 2-month follow-up period:* A detailed assessment of the patient's present functioning, including cognitive functioning, was carried out prior to the initiation of the intervention program. SS was assessed for his overall level of functioning using the Global Assessment of Functioning (GAF) scale of the DSM-IV [90]. The GAF is a single rating scale used for clinical assessment of a patient's overall level of functioning. The GAF requires the clinician to make a global assessment of a patient's current level of psychological, social, and occupational functioning. Scale values range from 1 to 100, and are divided into 10 equal intervals, e.g., 91–100, indicating the highest level of functioning, or 0–10, indicating the lowest level of functioning. The GAF is a revised version of the Global Assessment Scale [114] that was used to evaluate a patient's overall level of functioning on Axis V of the DSM-III-R.

**Table 7.1** Schedule for Cognitive Retraining Program—IPI (Hegde et al., 2007)

| Cognitive Ability | Week 1 | Week 2 | Week 3 | Week 4 | Week 5 | Week 6 |
|---|---|---|---|---|---|---|
| Attention | Letter cancellation Dictation | Letter cancellation Dictation | Letter cancellation | Letter cancellation With distraction (music) | Letter cancellation With distraction (music) | Letter cancellation With distraction (music) |
| Fluency | Verbal Fluency | Verbal Fluency | | | | |
| Information Processing | Grain sorting | Grain sorting | Grain sorting | Grain sorting With distraction (music) | Grain sorting With distraction (music) | Grain sorting With distraction (music) |
| Working Memory | Arithmetic Jumbled sentences | Arithmetic Jumbled sentences | | | | |
| Response Inhibition | Coloring | Coloring | Coloring | Coloring | Coloring Start–stop tasks | Coloring Start–stop tasks |
| Immediate Visual Memory | | Designs | Designs | Designs | Designs | Designs |
| Spatial Encoding | | 3 objects | 4 objects | 5 objects | 6 objects | |
| Set-Shifting | | | Beads categorization | Cards categorization | Cards categorization | Cards categorization |
| Planning | | | Planning a task | Planning a task | Motor set-shifting Essay writing | Motor set-shifting Essay writing |
| Comprehension of facial expressions | | | Naming the different emotional expression | Naming the different emotional expression | Naming the different emotional expression | |

Neurocognitive functions were assessed using a battery of neuropsychological tests. The scores on the neuropsychological tests were compared with norms appropriate to the subject's gender, age, and education. The normative data was derived from a group of 540 normal healthy volunteers [91]. The 15th percentile score (1 SD below the mean) was taken as the cutoff score (Heaton et al. [92]). Cutoff scores were then calculated for each group based on age, education, and gender. A deficit was defined as a test score falling below the 15th percentile [92]. The tests included in the battery were

| Tests | Neurocognitive function |
| --- | --- |
| Digit vigilance test [93] | Sustained attention |
| Color trails test [94] | Focused attention |
| Finger tapping test [95] | Motor speed |
| Digit symbol substitution [96] | Mental speed |
| Self-ordering pointing test [97] | Working memory |
| Stroop test [91] | Response inhibition |
| Tower of London [98] | Planning |
| WCST[99] | Concept formation and set-shifting ability |
| Rey's Auditory Verbal Learning Test (RAVLT) [100] | Verbal learning and memory |
| Rey Osterrieth Complex Figure Test [101] | Visual learning and memory |

*Brief Clinical History*: Patient SS, a 29-year-old male, diagnosed with paranoid schizophrenia per the ICD-10 criteria [1]. SS was unmarried, had education up to B.E. in electronics, from a lower socioeconomic status, urban background. SS had a family history of alcohol dependence syndrome in father and arthritis in mother. SS was the only son and had lost his father at the age of 16. Father died of jaundice and liver problems, ill health perhaps due to his excessive drinking habit. SS had illness history of 14 years with predominant symptoms such as abusive and aggressive behavior, poor personal hygiene, irrelevant speech, delusions of persecutions and reference, smiling to self, and abusive behavior. He had been treated as an inpatient for several months in the past. SS had significant negative symptomatology such as slowness in activities and lack of motivation. SS also reported concentration problems. He was on Sizopin 300 mg, on regular medication.

SS did not have a paid job. He had been going to an electronic goods repair shop near to his place. Patient carried out simple activities such as repairing very simple items under the supervision of the owner and assisting the owner in getting the necessary item. Each day the owner would give the patient enough money for his food and commuting charges. At home, the patient hardly took any responsibilities in performing daily household chores. SS experienced excessive drowsiness in the morning hours and thus would get up late in the morning. He had to be repeatedly reminded of tasks that he needed to perform. His mother would perform all the household chores including some of his activities such as washing his clothes.

Mother was the breadwinner of the family. She was 55 years old, educated up to 10th standard. After the demise of the father and the onset of the illness of SS, the family had suffered significant financial problems, sliding down from a middle to a lower socioeconomic status. She worked as a housemaid in the neighborhood. She suffered from arthritis since several years. Her understanding of the illness was limited and poor. She felt that it was the medications that were making him dull and slow in his overall functioning. She opined that termination of medications and getting the patient married would make him active and normal.

## Preintervention Assessment of the Patient

The neuropsychological assessment during the preintervention assessment revealed impairment in the areas of sustained attention, sustained involving perceptual tracking and simple sequencing, mental speed, psychomotor speed, working memory, set shifting, planning, visual learning, and memory.

The GAF score was 51, indicating a moderate level of impairment in overall functioning.

Figure 7.1 depicts the percentile score on each of the neuropsychological variables assessed at the preintervention, postintervention, and 2-month follow-up assessment.

## Preintervention Assessment of the Caregiver

The caregiver, the mother of the patient in this case, was assessed on the General Health Questionnaire-28 (GHQ-28) [115] and Burden Assessment Schedule (BAS)

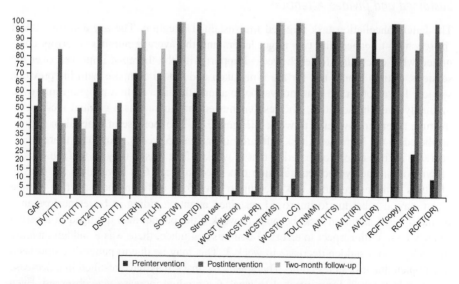

**Figure 7.1 Graph depicting the percentile score on each of the neuropsychological variable assessed on Pt.** SS at preintervention, postintervention, and at 2-month follow-up assessment period. GAF, global assessment of functioning score; DVT(TT), digital vigilance test (time taken in seconds); CTI(TT), CT2(TT), color trails test 1 and 2 (time taken in seconds); DSST(TT), digital symbol substitution test (time taken in seconds).

[102]. The mother of the patient had a score of 4 (cutoff score 4/5) on the GHQ. She reported poor health in the area of somatic symptoms, anxiety and insomnia, and depression. On the BAS, she obtained a score of 68, indicating that the experience of burden was fairly high. The specific areas of feelings of burden were physical and mental health of the caregiver, such as experiencing increased workload, feeling tired and exhausted, and frustration to some extent that improvement of patient was slow; in providing support to the patient, as the family's financial position was insufficient to take care of the patient, being forced to work to support the patient; in taking responsibility such as feeling responsible to meet the patient's financial needs, concern over patient's future financial situation, concern over family's financial situation that has worsened since the patient's illness; and lack of external support such as support from family.

# The Cognitive Remediation Program

SS started with the 6-week hospital-based cognitive remediation program soon after the preintervention assessments were completed. Readers are referred to the published manuscript for a detailed description of the cognitive remediation program [33].

## Attention

### Sustained and Divided Attention

The letter-cancellation task targeted the sustained attention. The average time taken (in seconds) to cancel the two target letters and the average number of errors committed were calculated for each week. Rapport with the therapist improved over the sessions. Patient would ask for the time taken and would compare with his previous session. It was observed that motivation to attend the intervention program improved gradually over the sessions. The results showed that there was a gradual increase in the time taken from week 1 to week 5 (Figure 7.2). The increase in time taken may be attributed to the increase in task difficulty over these 5 weeks. However, there was a decrease in time taken compared to that of week 5. The reason may be that the density of symbols in the symbol-cancellation task used in week 6 is lower than the density of letters in the cancellation task used up to week 5. In addition, the reduction of time taken may also be due to improved sustained attention aiding in better performance on the divided attention task, because in week 6 the patient also indulged in a verbal fluency task. With respect to errors of commission made, there was a sudden increase in week 2 and a sudden decrease in week 3. This may be due to patient's enthusiasm to complete the task in less time. Therapist's feedback may have resulted in a decrease in errors in week 3. From week 4 to week 6 a gradual increase was observed. Even though the density of symbols was less in week 6 as compared to the density of letters in week 5, there was an increase in errors committed. This may be due to patient concentrating on the verbal fluency task that was presented as a task targeting divided attention (Figure 7.3).

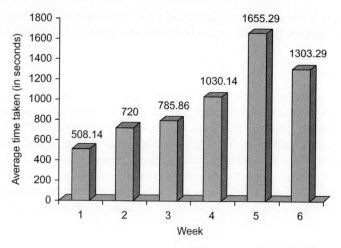

**Figure 7.2** Letter-cancellation task, average time taken in seconds.

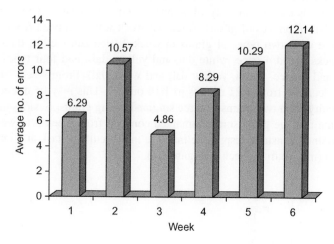

**Figure 7.3** Letter-cancellation task, average errors of omission.

## Focused Attention

The dictation task, wherein words were given for which patient had to write the spelling, was included in the week 1 and week 2 of the retraining program. This task targeted the focused attention. The difficulty level was decided, keeping in mind the patient's ability to spell difficult words. The average number of words correctly spelled in each week was calculated. In the first week, patient had an average score of 14.43 and in week 2, the score was 14. Though there was an increase in the difficulty of the words given for dictation from week 1 to 2, there was no substantial change in the scores, indicating an improvement in focused attention. Behavioral observation indicated that patient was able to focus his attention while performing the task. Patient was curious to know the correct spelling of those words that were wrongly spelled. Therapist did give the feedback, as this maintained the patient's motivation level.

### Verbal Fluency

The patient was observed to show interest in this task. Patient would initially start giving proper nouns, which was discouraged, and he was motivated to generate words other than names of persons and places. Patient was at times given feedback and hints to generate simple words used in everyday usage after the day's performance. The score on each day was the average number of words generated in 2 min for each of the two letters. An average score of the number of words generated for each week was also calculated. Though there has not been a significant increase in the number of words generated, there was a qualitative improvement in the nature of words generated.

### Information Processing

In the first week, the time taken to sort the two types of grains was noted down. In subsequent weeks, the quantity of grains sorted was measured in ounces. The average number of ounces of grains sorted per week was calculated from week 2 to week 6. There were two types of grains in week 2 (rice and methi), three types of grains in weeks 3 and 4 (rice, white dal, and yellow dal), and four types of grains in weeks 5 and 6 (rice, methi, yellow dal, and white dal). From week 2 to week 3 there was a decrease from 3.21 ounces to 1.14 ounces. This may be due to increase in task difficulty from two grains to three similar-looking grains. Besides an increase in week 4, the average grain sorted remained constant from week 5 to week 6. The quantity remained constant despite the increase in difficulty of task and introduction of distraction (music) from week 4 (Figure 7.4).

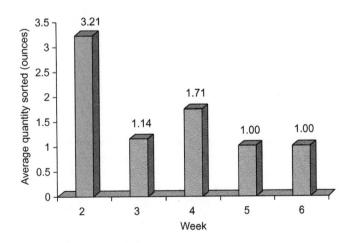

**Figure 7.4** Grain-sorting task, average quality sorted (ounces).

## Response Inhibition

Coloring a given design was the task given from week 1 to week 6, targeting the response inhibition function. For week 1 to week 4, the task was to color a square (14 cms). The difficulty of the task was increased by increasing the number of sections in the figure from 1 to 4 from week 1 to week 4. In weeks 5 and 6, drawings of fruits, flowers, house, etc., were included. The average time taken to color the given area per week was recorded (in seconds). The time taken to complete the task was observed to have increased gradually until week 1 to week 6 (Figure 7.5). The patient may have taken more time as the difficulty level of the task increased. Patient reported he enjoyed this task. In the first few sessions, patient had to be reminded of the quality of the work, such as even pressure on the pencil, evenness in coloring the whole area, and neatness. Patient expressed happiness in weeks 5 and 6 when meaningful drawings were introduced.

## Stop Tasks with Movements

This task targeted the function of response inhibition. The patient was made to perform a motor task such as clapping hands, lifting the arm, and letting it down. Therapist suddenly asked the patient to stop the motor task he had been performing. Initially, patient would not cease the task immediately; there would be a delay in following the start and stop signals given by the therapist. Patient was physically very well built and was overweight. In this task, patient was initially very slow and would try doing tasks with the minimum movements possible. When encouraged and given clues about various movements, he was able to perform the task.

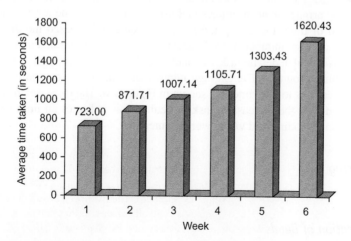

**Figure 7.5** Coloring task, average time taken (in seconds).

## Working Memory

### Arithmetic Problems

Arithmetic problems targeting the working memory component were included. Patient was given arithmetic problem having four numbers and an arithmetic formula. Patient had to give the final answer to the therapist. The average time taken per week (in seconds) and number of trials were recorded. The average time taken in week 1 was 27.47 s and in week 2 it was 37.73 s. A difference of 10 s was observed. The average number of trials taken was 1.53 in week 1 and 1.41 in week 2. There was no significant difference in the average time and in the average number of trials taken in week 1 and week 2. The therapist observed that patient was interested in doing this task. He would express his disappointment when he failed to get an answer right. Patient in his anxiety to get the answer in less time would fail to register the facts correctly. He was encouraged to get the facts (numbers and operations) correctly and not to ask for a second trial. The increased difficulty in task did not lead to increased number of trials or time taken.

### Jumbled Sentences

The patient was given the task of orally correcting a jumbled sentence and reporting the sentence in a grammatically correct manner. The average number of trials taken per week was recorded. The average number of trials taken in week 1 was 1.29 and in week 2 was 1.50. There was no significant change in the average number of trials from week 1 to week 2, though the difficulty of task had increased. Besides showing interest in the task, patient also was observed expressing disappointment when he made a mistake.

## Visual Working Memory

Spatial encoding and memory was targeted by this task, where patient was exposed to a particular arrangement of objects and asked to reproduce the arrangement after a brief period of time. Increasing the number of objects increased the difficulty of the task. The average number of trials taken to reproduce the arrangement correctly per week was calculated. The task was included from week 2 to week 5 of the cognitive retraining program. The average number of trials taken gradually increased from initial sessions to later ones, as shown in Figure 7.6. The increase appears to be less compared with the increase in task difficulty. This indicates an improvement in patient's visual encoding and visual working memory.

## Set Shifting

The function of set shifting was targeted using three different tasks.

### Categorization of Beads

Different varieties of beads were presented to the patient. In the first session, patient had to be given instructions in detail and no clue was given. In the first session, he

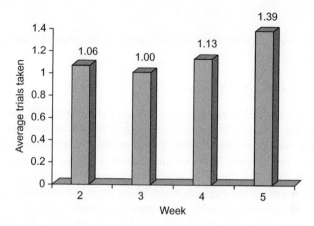

**Figure 7.6** Spatial encoding task, average trails taken.

started categorizing, and when the therapist posed questions he was able to get a clear understanding in to the task. Over the sessions he was able to come up with principles such as opaque, semiopaque, and transparent beads, which therapist had not recorded as a possible category. He would sometimes express the principle halfway through the categorization of the beads and ambivalence to categorizing the remaining beads, indicating that patient showed improved ability to categorize and form new concepts based on the rules of the tasks.

## Categorization of Cards

Two decks of playing cards were taken, with all the cards with faces removed. The patient responded to this task with interest. Patient was given thorough instructions before starting the task. Patient in the initial two to three sessions had difficulty guessing the principle the therapist had in mind. He was given hints and encouraged to think of the reason for the responses being incorrect. In week 5, the patient had to keep in mind a principle and the therapist would sort the cards. The patient was instructed to give feedback by saying "correct" or "incorrect," keeping in mind the principle given. Difficulty in getting newer principles and loosening of the principle that he started with was observed. It was observed by the end of 2 weeks that patient was able to think of new principles, such as the consecutive numbers to be placed in a category, alternating the color of the card and the number.

## Motor Set-Shifting Tasks

Patient was to indulge in a continuous pattern of motor tasks such as clapping, tapping hands, and various rhythmic tapping with hands. Once the patient was observed to be involved in the task, he was asked to suddenly change over to a different pattern of task. However, patient had difficulty in shifting over to a new task immediately. There were repetitions of the tasks. He was given feedback immediately and encouraged to shift to a new task.

## Planning

Planning ability was targeted using two different tasks: planning tasks of real-life situations and essay writing.

### Planning Task of Real-Life Situations

Patient was given a real-life situation such as preparing breakfast for two people, planning to go for a movie, and purchasing a gift for a friend within a budget of 200 rupees. The nature of steps involved to plan the given task decided the difficulty level of the task. Patient in the initial sessions was observed to report the steps involved very briefly. The therapist would pose questions, help patient report in detail, and help rearrange the steps involved. Many times the therapist would hypothesize certain consequences of having taken particular steps. It was observed this task targeted patient's problem-solving abilities along with planning. The topic for each day was chosen keeping in mind the patient's interests and hobbies. The therapist recorded the patient's responses on this task. Over the sessions it was observed that patient was able to narrate the steps involved in much detail.

### Essay Writing

In this task patient was given a topic and asked to write an essay on the given topic. He was also given information regarding the different components of the essay, such as the introduction, core material (body), and conclusions. Some of the topics were chosen keeping in mind the patient's interests, and some were general topics, for example, various electrical circuits, nature, Indian food, election, and money. Therapist would sometimes discuss and help patient generate much more information. He was observed to be interested in discussion. The content and flow of thought in the essay improved over sessions. Patient at times also showed interest in gathering information from other sources such as books or magazines and reported to the therapist in the following session.

### Visual Immediate Memory

The component of visual encoding and memory was targeted by the task involving designs. The patient was exposed to 10 designs with few components. Patient was asked to reproduce the design after a brief exposure. The average score per week was calculated. The scores indicate slight improvement as the training continued (Figure 7.7). Behavioral observation revealed that patient was very interested in this activity and he would count the correct ones at the end of each session. He would show emotional reaction such as disappointment, surprise, and happiness when the designs seemed difficult, challenging, or simple enough to obtain another score.

### Comprehension and Production of Emotions

This task was more interactive in nature. The therapist would express certain emotions via facial gestures, and patient was asked to identify the emotion expressed.

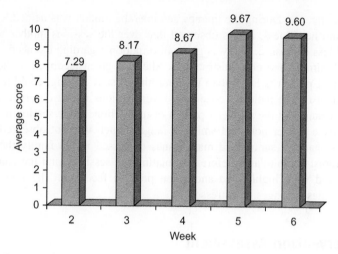

**Figure 7.7** Design task, average score.

Patient needed no clue to identify the gross emotions such as sadness, happiness, and anger. Later in week 3, patient was able to grasp subtle emotions such as disappointment, curiosity, surprise, and suspiciousness. At times therapist had to use simple dialogues while depicting the emotions. In week 4, the patient was asked to express various emotions through facial gestures during the session. Patient was observed to be very much interested and enthusiastic in performing the task. In week 5, therapist and patient collaboratively identified various situations, and patient was to express his reaction and emotions. Improvement and quickness in the patient in grasping the emotions expressed was observed.

## Family Intervention

Family intervention was initiated after the preintervention assessment. Mother of SS was observed to be highly critical of the patient and wanted the medications to be stopped immediately. Rapport was difficult to establish. She strongly believed that the medications were making him lethargic and amotivated. She was willing to attend the family session, though she was suffering from severe arthritis and had difficulty in commuting long distance. Her main expectation from the patient was to start earning his daily living and also to get married. Psychoeducation sessions were held to provide information regarding the nature of the illness. It was after five or six sessions, mother was able to accept what the therapist was telling her regarding the illness.

Activity scheduling was done for the patient. Mother, however, expected patient to start earning regularly but never expected him to do any household chores. She would feel sorry for patient and would even perform activities that patient was capable of doing. Activity scheduling was done and patient was motivated to carry out his day-to-day activities accordingly. Changes in mother's attitude toward the patient's ability to perform had changed and she seemed to let patient to do activities she never let him do earlier. These included activities such as buying groceries, collecting water, etc. During the therapy sessions the mother was helped to vent her problems and her illness. It was observed that over the sessions mother was much calmer and less distressed. She was given information regarding the need to instruct patient with simple and clear instructions. She was given feedback on her critical comments that patient is lazy, often nagging him to start earning, could have a detrimental effect on the patient's condition. Over sessions it was observed that there were some changes in the mother's pattern of interaction. In the session mother was able to enjoy a lighter note and smile or laugh, which was not observed initially. Mother was made to summarize main issues discussed in the family therapy sessions. Therapist recapitulated before terminating the sessions, and the changes that were observed were highlighted and given positive feedback. The importance of maintaining these changes was stressed.

## Postintervention Assessment

There was improvement and normalization in sustained attention, psychomotor speed, response inhibition, working memory, set shifting, planning, verbal learning, and visual learning and memory. Verbal memory declined from the preassessment period, though it remained in the nondeficient level.

### 2-Month Follow-Up Assessment

Mental speed that was in the normal range improved further. Sustained attention, response inhibition, and working memory declined in the postintervention period, though it continued to remain in the normal range and remained higher than in the preintervention period.

### Global Functioning of the Patient at Postintervention and at 2-Month Follow-Up Period

At postintervention the GAF score was 67, which indicated improvement in overall functioning of the patient from preintervention period. At 2-month follow-up the score was 61. The score had decreased from the postretraining assessment (67), though it remained at a higher level compared to the preintervention level of functioning, indicating maintenance of improvement despite cessation of regular intervention sessions.

### Postintervention Assessment of the Caregiver

At the end of 12 sessions of family intervention, caregiver was reassessed on the GHQ and the BAS. On the GHQ, the postintervention score indicated general health status was good. On the BAS, she obtained a score of 47. The score during the preintervention assessment on this scale was 68. This indicates a reduction in the feeling of burden in taking care of the family member with schizophrenia. Perceived burden was less in aspects such as concern over patient's future financial status and frustration due to slow improvement. Mother reported that drowsiness in patient during the morning hours continued; however, she had stopped waking him up or nagging. She was happy that patient had improved his personal hygiene and was performing certain household chores that helped her, such as washing clothes and purchasing groceries. Mother had stopped asking therapist about stopping of medications; instead, she would ask if the dosage could be reduced over time.

## 2-Month Follow-Up Assessment of the Caregiver

At the end of 2-month follow-up session of family intervention, caregiver was reassessed on the GHQ and the BAS. Mother obtained a score of 3, indicating that the general health was good. On the BAS she obtained a score of 53. The score during the postintervention assessment on this scale had been 47. This indicates an increase in the feeling of burden from the postintervention assessment, though it was lower compared to the preintervention assessment of 68. The areas of concern remained unchanged.

## Summary

The IPI was a hospital-based 6-week program. The cognitive remediation program included paper-and-pencil and tasks based on materials used in day-to-day functioning that did not add much to the treatment cost. The results were promising. The intervention showed that a 6-week program was effective in improving neurocognitive functions such as attention, psychomotor speed, response inhibition, and executive functions in chronically ill patients. Careful examination of the gradual yet positive changes in patient's interaction with the therapist during the intervention program indicated improvement in motivation. This also was reflected in patient's compliance to medication. Maintenance of improvement even 2 months after completion of the intervention proves further that cognitive remediation in schizophrenia is possible and must be an integral part of treatment program. In the case illustrated in the text and two other patients who underwent this intervention program, all were gainfully employed during the postintervention and follow-up period. Although insight or motivation were not quantitatively measured using a standardized tool in this case, a definite improvement in motivation was observed within few sessions after initiation of the cognitive retraining program. Perhaps there is a cascading effect of improvement of basic cognitive functions onto the higher cognitive functions such as executive functions and even insight. A gradual increase in task difficulty and a well-planned cognitive remediation program are the keys to success.

Family intervention proved to be beneficial for family members of the chronically ill schizophrenia patients. It is important to address various issues the primary caregivers have, such as concerns related to the future of the illness, future plans of the patient, and also feelings of burden. The caregiver experienced burden, especially due to the concerns that families expressed regarding the patient's future and their expectations of the patient in the of social and occupational domains of functioning.

It was observed that the family members needed psychoeducation regarding the nature, etiology, treatment options, and course and outcome of the illness. Although the scores on perceived burden did not change significantly from pre- to postintervention or from postintervention to the 2-month follow-up period, the caregiver reported that the intervention sessions helped her reexamine the situation, gain better understanding of the patient's illness, and feel more in control. One should remember that this patient was chronically ill and it would be impractical to believe that the objective feelings of burden would be changed in this short period.

Noh and Avison (1987) [116] have reported that subjective burden rather than objective burden was linked to psychological well-being. The aspects observed in this study are similar to those of Oldrigde and Hughes (1992) [117], who assessed the level of distress and burden in the primary caregivers of patients with chronic schizophrenia. They reported that 36% of the caregivers qualified for caseness on the GHQ and the Hospital Anxiety and Depression Scale (HADS). Greater degree of distress was associated with negative symptoms in patients, and objective burden was significantly correlated with the anxiety and insomnia subscale of the GHQ and anxiety and insomnia subscale and depression on the HADS. Hatfield and Lefley (2000) [118] in their study have shown that caregivers experienced intense anxiety about the future of the ill family member, lack of knowledge of how to plan, lack of financial resources, patient's refusal to use available resources, and resistance to change were cited as barriers that the caregivers faced. A study carried out by Gidron (1991) [119] reported that caregivers expressed concerns regarding the future of the patient and the family. The concerns the families mainly revolve around the future and the expectations they have of the patient, as well as the burden due to various aspects involved in taking care of patient with schizophrenia.

The IPI, however, is quite time- and labor-intensive from the therapist's point of view. This is a serious impediment to wide application of the intervention program. In India, with very few trained psychologists and neuropsychologists, a wide application of the IPI would be difficult. The current approach to cognitive remediation, although effective, is time consuming and therefore not cost-effective.

## Cognitive Remediation in the Early Phase of the Illness

Despite the fact that cognitive deficits are present prior to the onset of illness and persist after remission of the psychotic symptoms, very few studies have targeted remediation of cognitive deficits as part of the treatment at the onset of the illness [73,103,104]. Since cognitive deficits and social functioning are related, improving cognitive functions at the onset of the illness would have a beneficial effect on the course and outcome of the illness. Longitudinal studies suggest that the most devastating clinical progression in patients with schizophrenia occurs within the first 5 years from the time of onset. Early stages of the illness also reflect an active pathophysiological process that can produce enduring cognitive and functional impairment in patients and reduce their capacity to respond to treatment [105]. It is plausible that early intervention could have the potential to reverse some of the disability associated with the illness. Treatment introduced from the early stages of the illness may prevent long-term morbidity that tragically affects the lives of patients and their families and results in a great economic burden to society.

A home-based cognitive remediation program developed for patients in the first phase of schizophrenia has shown promising results in improving cognitive functions as well decreasing negative symptoms. A randomized controlled study to examine the effectiveness of this 2-month-long, home-based cognitive retraining program together with treatment as usual—TAU (psychoeducation and drug therapy)—was carried out on neuropsychological functions, psychopathology, and global functioning in patients with FES as well as on psychological health and perception of level of family distress in their caregivers [81]. Forty-five FES patients were randomly assigned to either treatment group, who received home-based cognitive retraining along with TAU ($n = 22$) or to control group who received TAU alone ($n = 23$). Patients and caregivers received psychoeducation. Patients and one of their caregivers were assessed on the above parameters at baseline, postassessment (2-month), and at 6-month follow-up assessment. This is the first study that has developed and examined the effect of home-based retraining program in FES patients. The significant interaction effect has shown that the addition of cognitive retraining to TAU led to improvement in executive functions such as divided attention, planning, concept formation, and set-shifting ability following treatment. Effect sizes were large (Cohen's $d = 0.99$), although the sample size was small. Further, the improvement had been sustained for 6 months even though treatment had ceased. The improved cognition in the treatment group cannot be attributed to practice on the neuropsychological tests, as the control group also underwent the pre-, post-, and follow-up assessments.

A home-based cognitive retraining program involves tasks that can be performed by the patient himself/herself with less monitoring by a family member would reduce the financial and personal burden of visiting the hospital frequently. The clinician would be able to treat a large number of patients in a given time frame. The multimodal intervention program would then be a cost-effective treatment for schizophrenia. Despite the lack of trained clinicians to monitor daily cognitive retraining sessions, the program improved cognitive functions such as attention, planning and concept formation, and set-shifting ability in FES patients.

The combination of drug treatment and psychoeducation along with cognitive retraining has been shown to benefit patients. Studies have indicated that responsiveness to social skills training procedures was predicted by pretreatment verbal memory, fluency, and reasoning ability [48]. In this case, introducing cognitive retraining at the very beginning of the treatment program and consequent changes in domains of attention and executive functions has probably benefited patients in more than one way. The advantage may have been in bringing about an insight into the illness, as changes in executive functions lead to better insight. Improvement in cognitive functions has augmented benefits from psychoeducation sessions. Decrease in negative symptoms has been associated with improved social functioning and in aspects of social perception and performance [106]. Along with this, simultaneous changes in the understanding of the illness by caregivers probably has led to lower stress levels in the family environment. Also, improved cognitive functions may have contributed to improvement in patients' ability to handle stress in day-to-day functioning, for example, in ability to handle deadlines in work setting. The psychoeducational program, especially in the FES group, has been shown to help caregivers play a supportive, constructive role in the management of the illness. In the treatment group, improved cognition could have enhanced the patient's ability to process information from the environment and react appropriately, thereby modulating the perception of the nature of the rewards obtained from the environment. A positive feedback loop may be set up whereby appropriate reaction by the patient could lead to enhanced environmental rewards, which in turn motivates the patient further, thereby leading to improved social interactions. This interaction between the environment and the individual's reaction has activated the response–reward network, which is otherwise known to be impaired in schizophrenia patients.

Improved cognitive functioning might have improved occupational functioning, leading to increased social stimulation. The caregivers who had better understanding of the illness following the psychoeducation sessions may have helped in maintaining a supportive environment. When a patient and caregivers visit the hospital in the initial phase of the illness, the family has little knowledge of the causes, symptoms, and management of the illness. Tolerance toward changes in the patient's behavior and symptoms presented will be fairly high. The caregivers who were chiefly parents and spouses had not reached the level of distress that is generally observed when the chronicity of illness and illness duration was longer. It is known from previous studies that improving caregivers' knowledge about the illness leads to a decrease in relapse and rehospitalization [107,108]. The increased knowledge gained through psychoeducation may have improved their psychological health as well as resulted in a decrease in perceived level of distress. It is possible that psychoeducational programs for caregivers bring about change in attitude [109]. The attitude of family members toward the ill member is known to have a significant influence on the patient's ability to carry out his responsibilities in general, as reflected in improvement in global functioning. Hence the changes in caregivers' understanding of the illness may have in turn contributed to adherence to treatment. Family environment is an important factor influencing the course and outcome of the illness. Patients with schizophrenia and their families benefit from education and feedback regarding the illness, prognosis, and treatment. The addition of psychoeducation to the treatment program has shown significant reduction in relapse and readmission rates and improved family well-being [86].

This understanding of the interaction between the improvement in cognitive function, improvement in understanding of the illness condition by patients and caregivers, compliance to treatment, reduced stress level, and the interaction among all these factors can be depicted as in Figure 7.8.

## Summary and Future Directions

Deficits in neurocognitive functions are a manifestation of the neuropathology and an important predictor of outcome in schizophrenia. Cognitive deficits have been known to limit long-term outcome. They affect work performance, community

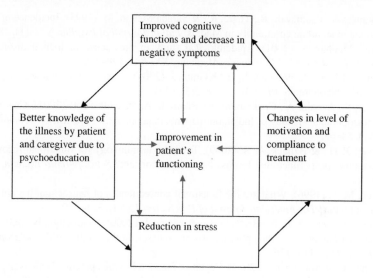

**Figure 7.8** Depicting the interaction between targets of treatment program and global functioning.

functioning, social problem solving, and social skill acquisition, as well as ability to benefit from other psychosocial treatment methods. The increasing awareness of the central role of cognitive deficits in schizophrenia has fostered considerable interest in the prospects of cognitive rehabilitation. Maintenance of improved cognitive functions and generalization of improved cognitive functions to day-to-day functioning and overall functioning have been a challenge for clinicians across the globe. Despite the fact that cognitive deficits are present prior to the onset of illness and persist after remission of the psychotic symptoms, very few studies have targeted remediation of cognitive deficits as part of the treatment at the onset of the illness. The effectiveness of cognitive remediation programs has been seen chiefly in chronically ill patients, with only a handful in the early phase of the illness. Treatment introduced from the early stages of the illness may prevent the long-term morbidity that tragically affects the lives of patients and their families and results in a great economic burden to society. Cognitive remediation should be treated as an important treatment modality at the very onset of this debilitating illness. It is quite evident from studies that there is a need to integrate cognitive remediation with other treatment programs such as pharmacological management, psychoeducation, family intervention, and social skills training for an effective outcome in this illness.

# References

[1] WHO, (1992). *The ICD-10 diagnostic classification of mental and behavioural disorders.* Geneva: World Health Organization.
[2] APA, (1993). *Diagnostic and statistical manual of mental fisorders.* Washington, DC: American Psychiatric Association.

[3] Rajkumar, S., Padmavati, R., Thara, R., & Sarada Menon, M. (1993). Incidence of schizophrenia in an urban community in Madras. *Indian Journal of Psychiatry, 35*(1), 18–21.

[4] Murali Madhav, S. (2001). Epideiological study of prevalence of mental disorders in India. *Indian Journal of Community Medicine, XXVI*(4), 198–200.

[5] Saha, S., Chant, D., Welham, J., & McGrath, J. (2005). A systematic review of the prevalence of schizophrenia. *PLoS Medicine, 2*(5), e141.

[6] Grover, S., Avasthi, A., Chakrabarti, S., Bhansali, A., & Kulhara, P. (2005). Cost of care of schizophrenia: A study of Indian out-patient attenders. *Acta Psychiatrica Scandinavica, 112*(1), 54–63.

[7] Harvey, P. D., & Bellack, A. S. (2009). Toward a terminology for functional recovery in Schizophrenia: Is functional Remission a viable concept? *Schizophrenia Bulletin, 35*(2), 300–306.

[8] Green, M. F. (1996). What are the functional consequences of neurocognitive deficits in schizophrenia? *The American Journal of Psychiatry, 153*(3), 321–330.

[9] Green, M. F., Kern, R. S., Braff, D. L., & Mintz, J. (2000). Neurocognitive deficits and functional outcome in schizophrenia: Are we measuring the "right stuff"? *Schizophrenia Bulletin, 26*(1), 119–136.

[10] Sharma, T., & Antonova, L. (2003). Cognitive function in schizophrenia. Deficits, functional consequences, and future treatment. *The Psychiatric Clinics of North America, 26*(1), 25–40.

[11] Buckley, P. F. (1998). Preface. *The Psychiatric Clinics of North America*(21), xi–xiii.

[12] Flashman, L. A., & Green, M. F. (2004). Review of cognition and brain structure in schizophrenia: Profiles, longitudinal course, and effects of treatment. *The Psychiatric Clinics of North America, 27*(1), 1–18. vii.

[13] Saykin, A. J., Shtasel, D. L., Gur, R. E., Kester, D. B., Mozley, L. H., Stafiniak, P., et al. (1994). Neuropsychological deficits in neuroleptic naive patients with first-episode schizophrenia. *Archives of General Psychiatry, 51*(2), 124–131.

[14] Censits, D. M., Ragland, J. D., Gur, R. C., & Gur, R. E. (1997). Neuropsychological evidence supporting a neurodevelopmental model of schizophrenia: A longitudinal study. *Schizophrenia Research, 24*(3), 289–298.

[15] Riley, E. M., McGovern, D., Mockler, D., Doku, V. C., O'Ceallaigh, O. C., Fannon, D. G., et al. (2000). Neuropsychological functioning in first-episode psychosis--evidence of specific deficits. *Schizophrenia Research, 43*(1), 47–55.

[16] Hoff, A. L., Riordan, H., O'Donnell, D. W., Morris, L., & DeLisi, L. E. (1992). Neuropsychological functioning of first-episode schizophreniform patients. *The American Journal of Psychiatry, 149*(7), 898–903.

[17] Bilder, R. M., Goldman, R. S., Robinson, D., Reiter, G., Bell, L., Bates, J. A., et al. (2000). Neuropsychology of first-episode schizophrenia: Initial characterization and clinical correlates. *The American Journal of Psychiatry, 157*(4), 549–559.

[18] Nelson, E. B., Sax, K. W., & Strakowski, S. M. (1998). Attentional performance in patients with psychotic and nonpsychotic major depression and schizophrenia. *The American Journal of Psychiatry, 155*(1), 137–139.

[19] Smith, G. L., Large, M. M., Kavanagh, D. J., Karayanidis, F., Barrett, N. A., Michie, P. T., et al. (1998). Further evidence for a deficit in switching attention in schizophrenia. *Journal of Abnormal Psychology, 107*(3), 390–398.

[20] Cadenhead, K. S., Geyer, M. A., Butler, R. W., Perry, W., Sprock, J., & Braff, D. L. (1997). Information processing deficits of schizophrenia patients: Relationship to clinical ratings, gender and medication status. *Schizophrenia Research, 28*(1), 51–62.

[21] Nestor, P. G., Akdag, S. J., O'Donnell, B. F., Niznikiewicz, M., Law, S., Shenton, M. E., et al. (1998). Word recall in schizophrenia: A connectionist model. *The American Journal of Psychiatry, 155*(12), 1685–1690.

[22] Huron, C., Danion, J. M., Giacomoni, F., Grange, D., Robert, P., & Rizzo, L. (1995). Impairment of recognition memory with, but not without, conscious recollection in schizophrenia. *The American Journal of Psychiatry, 152*(12), 1737–1742.

[23] Pantelis, C., Barber, F. Z., Barnes, T. R., Nelson, H. E., Owen, A. M., & Robbins, T. W. (1999). Comparison of set-shifting ability in patients with chronic schizophrenia and frontal lobe damage. *Schizophrenia Research, 37*(3), 251–270.

[24] Morris, R. G., Rushe, T., Woodruffe, P. W., & Murray, R. M. (1995). Problem solving in schizophrenia: A specific deficit in planning ability. *Schizophrenia Research, 14*(3), 235–246.

[25] Keshavan, M. S., Rabinowitz, J., DeSmedt, G., Harvey, P. D., & Schooler, N. (2004). Correlates of insight in first episode psychosis. *Schizophrenia Research, 70*(2–3), 187–194.

[26] Braff, D. L. (1993). Information processing and attention dysfunctions in schizophrenia. *Schizophrenia Bulletin, 19*(2), 233–259.

[27] Greig, T. C., Bryson, G. J., & Bell, M. D. (2004). Theory of mind performance in schizophrenia: Diagnostic, symptom, and neuropsychological correlates. *The Journal of Nervous and Mental Disease, 192*(1), 12–18.

[28] Rao, S. L. (2004). Cognitive dysfunction and cognitive remediation in schizophrenia. In: MKMnSH Nizamie (Ed.), *Current developments in schizophrenia.* Allied Publishers Pvt. Ltd.

[29] Ayres, A. M., Busatto, G. F., Menezes, P. R., Schaufelberger, M. S., Coutinho, L., Murray, R. M., et al. (2007). Cognitive deficits in first-episode psychosis: A population-based study in Sao Paulo, Brazil. *Schizophrenia Research, 90*(1–3), 338–343.

[30] Srinivasan, L., Thara, R., & Tirupati, S. N. (2005). Cognitive dysfunction and associated factors in patients with chronic schizophrenia. *Indian Journal of Psychiatry, 47*(3), 139–143.

[31] Ananthanarayanan, C., Janakiramaiah, N., Gangadhar, B., Vittal, S., Anrade, C., & Kumaraiah, V. (1993). Visual information processing deficits clinical remitted outpatient schizophrenics. *Indian Journal of Psychiatry, 35*, 27–30.

[32] John, P., Khanna, S., & Mukundan, C. (2001). Relationship between psychopathological dimensions and performance on frontal lobe tests in schizophrenia. *Indian Journal of Psycholoical Medicine, 24*, 19–26.

[33] Hegde, S., Rao, S. L., & Raguram, A. (2007). Integrated psychological internvention for schizophrenia. *International Journal of Psyxhosocial Rehabilitation, 11*(2), 5–18.

[34] Hegde, S., Thirthalli, J., Rao, S. L., Raguram, A., Gangadhar, B. (2008). Cognitive deficits and its relation with psychopathology and global functionoing in first episode schizophrenia.

[35] Kay, S. R., Fiszbein, A., & Opler, L. A. (1987). The positive and negative syndrome scale (PANSS) for schizophrenia. *Schizophrenia Bulletin, 13*(2), 261–276.

[36] WHO. (2002). WHODAS II. <http://wwwwhoint/icidh/whodas/> Accessed 05.09.04.

[37] Krishnadas, R., Moore, B., Nayak, A., & Patel, R. (2007). Relationship of cognitive function in patients with schizophrenia in remission to disability: A cross-sectional study in an Indian sample. *Annals of General Psychiatry, 6*, 19.

[38] Gold, J. M., & Harvey, P. D. (1993). Cognitive deficits in schizophrenia. *The Psychiatric Clinics of North America, 16*(2), 295–312.

[39] Goldberg, T. E., David, A. S., & Gold, J. M. (2003). Neurocognitive deficits in schizophrenia. In S. R. Hirsch, & D. Weinberger (Eds.), *Schizophrenia (pp. 168–687)* (2nd ed.). Massachusetts: Blackwell Science Limited.

[40] Fallon, J. H., Opole, I. O., & Potkin, S. G. (2003). The neuroanatomy of schizophrenia: Circuitry and neurotransmitter systems. *Clinical Neuroscience Research, 3*(2), 77–107.

[41] John, J. P. (2009). Fronto-temporal dysfunction in schizophrenia: A selective review. *Indian Journal of Psychiatry, 51*(3), 180–190.

[42] Padmavati, R. (2004). Neuroimaging in schizophrenia. In M. K. Mandal, & H. S. Nizamie (Eds.), *Current developments in schizophrenia (pp. 3–20).* Allied Publishers Pvt Ltd.

[43] Venkatasubramanian, G. (2010). Neuroanatomical correlates of psychopathology in antipsychotic-naive schizhophrenia. *Indian Journal of Psychiatry, 52*(1), 28–36.

[44] Bellack, A. S., Sayers, M., Mueser, K. T., & Bennett, M. (1994). Evaluation of social problem solving in schizophrenia. *Journal of Abnormal Psychology, 103*(2), 371–378.

[45] Bellack, A. S., Gold, J. M., & Buchanan, R. W. (1999). Cognitive rehabilitation for schizophrenia: Problems, prospects, and strategies. *Schizophrenia Bulletin, 25*(2), 257–274.

[46] McGurk, S. R., Moriarty, P. J., Harvey, P. D., Parrella, M., White, L., & Davis, K. L. (2000). The longitudinal relationship of clinical symptoms, cognitive functioning, and adaptive life in geriatric schizophrenia. *Schizophrenia Research, 42*(1), 47–55.

[47] Twamley, E. W., Doshi, R. R., Nayak, G. V., Palmer, B. W., Golshan, S., Heaton, R. K., et al. (2002). Generalized cognitive impairments, ability to perform everyday tasks, and level of independence in community living situations of older patients with psychosis. *The American Journal of Psychiatry, 159*(12), 2013–2020.

[48] Silverstein, S. M., Schenkel, L. S., Valone, C., & Nuernberger, S. W. (1998). Cognitive deficits and psychiatric rehabilitation outcomes in schizophrenia. *The Psychiatric Quarterly, 69*(3), 169–191.

[49] Bell, M. D., & Bryson, G. (2001). Work rehabilitation in schizophrenia: Does cognitive impairment limit improvement? *Schizophrenia Bulletin, 27*(2), 269–279.

[50] Weickert, T., & Goldberg, T. E., (2000). The course of cognitive impairment in patients with schizophrenia. In P. D. H. Tonmoy Sharma (Ed.), *Cognition in schizophrenia (pp. 3–15).* Oxford University Press.

[51] Flesher, S. (1990). Cognitive habilitation in schizophrenia: A theoretical review and model of treatment. *Neuropsychology Review, 1*(3), 223–246.

[52] Martindale, B. V., Mueser, K. T., Kuipers, E., Sensky, T., & Green, L. (2003). Psychological treatments for schizophrenia. In R. S. Hrisch, & D. Weinberger (Eds.), *Schizophrenia (pp. 657–687).* Blackwell Publishers.

[53] Rao, S. L. (Ed.). (1990). *Cognitive retraining. 3rd course in neurobiology for PGS in clinical neuroscience.* National Institute of Metal Health and NeuroSciences, (NIMHANS).

[54] Twamley, E. W., Jeste, D. V., & Bellack, A. S. (2003). A review of cognitive training in schizophrenia. *Schizophrenia Bulletin, 29*(2), 359–382.

[55] Goldberg, T. E., Weinberger, D. R., Berman, K. F., Pliskin, N. H., & Podd, M. H. (1987). Further evidence for dementia of the prefrontal type in schizophrenia? A controlled study of teaching the Wisconsin Card Sorting Test. *Archives of General Psychiatry, 44*(11), 1008–1014.

[56] Kurtz, M. M., Moberg, P. J., Gur, R. C., & Gur, R. E. (2001). Approaches to cognitive remediation of neuropsychological deficits in schizophrenia: A review and meta-analysis. *Neuropsychology Review, 11*(4), 197–210.

[57] Wykes, T., & van der Gaag, M. (2001). Is it time to develop a new cognitive therapy for psychosis–cognitive remediation therapy (CRT)? *Clinical Psychology Review, 21*(8), 1227–1256.

[58] Bellack, A. S., Mueser, K. T., Morrison, R. L., Tierney, A., & Podell, K. (1990). Remediation of cognitive deficits in schizophrenia. *The American Journal of Psychiatry, 147*(12), 1650–1655.

[59] Young, D. A., & Freyslinger, M. G. (1995). Scaffolded instruction and the remediation of Wisconsin Card Sorting Test deficits in chronic schizophrenia. *Schizophrenia Research, 16*(3), 199–207.

[60] Bellack, A. S., Blanchard, J. J., Murphy, P., & Podell, K. (1996). Generalization effects of training on the Wisconsin Card Sorting Test for schizophrenia patients. *Schizophrenia Research, 19*(2–3), 189–194.

[61] Summerfelt, A. T., Alphs, L. D., Wagman, A. M., Funderburk, F. R., Hierholzer, R. M., & Strauss, M. E. (1991). Reduction of perseverative errors in patients with schizophrenia using monetary feedback. *Journal of Abnormal Psychology, 100*(4), 613–616.

[62] Benedict, R. H., Harris, A. E., Markow, T., McCormick, J. A., Nuechterlein, K. H., & Asarnow, R. F. (1994). Effects of attention training on information processing in schizophrenia. *Schizophrenia Bulletin, 20*(3), 537–546.

[63] Medalia, A., Aluma, M., Tryon, W., & Merriam, A. E. (1998). Effectiveness of attention training in schizophrenia. *Schizophrenia Bulletin, 24*(1), 147–152.

[64] Bell, M., Bryson, G., & Wexler, B. E. (2003). Cognitive remediation of working memory deficits: Durability of training effects in severely impaired and less severely impaired schizophrenia. *Acta Psychiatrica Scandinavica, 108*(2), 101–109.

[65] van der Gaag, M., Kern, R. S., van den Bosch, R. J., & Liberman, R. P. (2002). A controlled trial of cognitive remediation in schizophrenia. *Schizophrenia Bulletin, 28*(1), 167–176.

[66] Wexler, B. E., Hawkins, K. A., Rounsaville, B., Anderson, M., Sernyak, M. J., & Green, M. F. (1997). Normal neurocognitive performance after extended practice in patients with schizophrenia. *Schizophrenia Research, 26*(2–3), 173–180.

[67] Wykes, T., Reeder, C., Corner, J., Williams, C., & Everitt, B. (1999). The effects of neurocognitive remediation on executive processing in patients with schizophrenia. *Schizophrenia Bulletin, 25*(2), 291–307.

[68] Hogarty, G. E., Flesher, S., Ulrich, R., Carter, M., Greenwald, D., Pogue-Geile, M., et al. (2004). Cognitive enhancement therapy for schizophrenia: Effects of a 2-year randomized trial on cognition and behavior. *Archives of General Psychiatry, 61*(9), 866–876.

[69] McGurk, S. R., & Mueser, K. T. (2004). Cognitive functioning, symptoms, and work in supported employment: A review and heuristic model. *Schizophrenia Research, 70*(2–3), 147–173.

[70] Bell, M., Bryson, G., Greig, T., Corcoran, C., & Wexler, B. E. (2001). Neurocognitive enhancement therapy with work therapy: Effects on neuropsychological test performance. *Archives of General Psychiatry, 58*(8), 763–768.

[71] Kurtz, M. M., Seltzer, J. C., Shagan, D. S., Thime, W. R., & Wexler, B. E. (2007). Computer-assisted cognitive remediation in schizophrenia: What is the active ingredient? *Schizophrenia Research, 89*(1–3), 251–260.

[72] Kern, R. S., Green, M. F., & Goldstein, M. J. (1995). Modification of performance on the span of apprehension, a putative marker of vulnerability to schizophrenia. *Journal of Abnormal Psychology, 104*(2), 385–389.

[73] Wykes, T., Newton, E., Landau, S., Rice, C., Thompson, N., & Frangou, S. (2007). Cognitive remediation therapy (CRT) for young early onset patients with schizophrenia: An exploratory randomized controlled trial. *Schizophrenia Research, 94*(1–3), 221–230.

[74] Brenner, H. D., Hodel, B., Roder, V., & Corrigan, P. (1992). Treatment of cognitive dysfunctions and behavioral deficits in schizophrenia. *Schizophrenia Bulletin, 18*(1), 21–26.

[75] Hogarty, G. E., & Flesher, S. (1999). Developmental theory for a cognitive enhancement therapy of schizophrenia. *Schizophrenia Bulletin, 25*(4), 677–692.

[76] Bell, M., Bryson, G., Greig, T., Corcoran, C., & Wexler, B. E. (2001). Neurocognitive enhancement therapy with work therapy: Effects on neuropsychological test performance. *Archives of General Psychiatry, 58*(8), 763–768.

[77] Delahunty, A., Morice, R., & Frost, B. (1993). Specific cognitive flexibility rehabilitation in schizophrenia. *Psychological Medicine, 23*(1), 221–227.

[78] Medalia, A., & Freilich, B. (2008). The neuropsychological educational approach to cognitive remediation (NEAR) model: Practice principles and outcome studies. *American Journal of Psychiatric Rehabilitation, 11*(2), 123–143.

[79] McGurk, S. R., Twamley, E. W., Sitzer, D. I., McHugo, G. J., & Mueser, K. T. (2007). A meta-analysis of cognitive remediation in schizophrenia. *The American Journal of Psychiatry, 164*(12), 1791–1802.

[80] Suslow, T., Schonauer, K., & Arolt, V. (2001). Attention training in the cognitive rehabilitation of schizophrenic patients: A review of efficacy studies. *Acta Psychiatrica Scandinavica, 103*(1), 15–23.

[81] Hegde, S., Rao, S. L., Raguram, A., & Gangadhar, B. N. (2011). Addition of home-based cognitive retraining to treatment as usual in first episode schizophrenia patients: A randomized controlled study. *Indian Journal of Psychiatry, 53*(4), 378–385.

[82] Srinivasan, T. N., & Thara, R. (2002). At issue: Management of medication noncompliance in schizophrenia by families in India. *Schizophrenia Bulletin, 28*(3), 531–535.

[83] Patel, V., Farooq, S., & Thara, R. (2007). What is the best approach to treating schizophrenia in developing countries? *PLOS Medicine, 4*(6) 0963–0996.

[84] Mueser, K. T., & Gingerich, S. L. (1994). *Coping with schizophrenia: A guide for families*. Oakland, CA: New Harbinger Publications.

[85] Braff, D. L., Heaton, R., Kuck, J., Cullum, M., Moranville, J., Grant, I., et al. (1991). The generalized pattern of neuropsychological deficits in outpatients with chronic schizophrenia with heterogeneous Wisconsin Card Sorting Test results. *Archives of General Psychiatry, 48*(10), 891–898.

[86] Dixon, L., Adams, C., & Lucksted, A. (2000). Update on family psychoeducation for schizophrenia. *Schizophrenia Bulletin, 26*(1), 5–20.

[87] Dixon, L., McFarlane, W. R., Lefley, H., Lucksted, A., Cohen, M., Falloon, I., et al. (2001). Evidence-based practices for services to families of people with psychiatric disabilities. *Psychiatric Services, 52*(7), 903–910.

[88] Bellack, A. S., Haas, G. L., Schooler, N. R., & Flory, J. D. (2000). Effects of behavioural family management on family communication and patient outcomes in schizophrenia. *The British Journal of Psychiatry, 177*, 434–439.

[89] Xiong, W., Phillips, M. R., Hu, X., Wang, R., Dai, Q., Kleinman, J., et al. (1994). Family-based intervention for schizophrenic patients in China. A randomised controlled trial. *The British Journal of Psychiatry, 165*(2), 239–247.

[90] APA, (1994). *Diagnostic and statistical manual of mental disorders*. Washington, DC: American Psychiatric Association.

[91] Rao, S. L., Subbakrishna, D. K., & Gopukumar, K. (2004). *NIMHANS neuropsycholoy battery-2004*. Banglaore: NIMHANS Publication.

[92] Heaton, R. K., Grant, I., Nelson, B., White, D. A., Kirson, D., & Atkinson, H. J. (1995). The HNRC500-neuropsychology of HIV infection at different disease stages. *Journal of the International Neuropsychological Society, 1*, 231–251.

[93] Lezak, M. D. (1995). *Neuropsychological assessment* (3rd ed.). New York: Oxford University Press.

[94] D'Elia, L. F., Satz, P., Uchiyama, C. L., & White, T. (1996). *Color trails test*. U S A: Psychological Assessment Resources Inc.

[95] Spreen, O., & Strauss, E. (1998). *A compendium of neuropsychological tests: Administration, norms and commentary* (2nd ed.). New York: Oxford University Press.

[96] Wechsler, D. (1981). *WAIS-R manual*. New York: The Psychological Corporation.

[97] Petrides, M., & Milner, B. (1982). Deficits on patient ordered tasks after frontal and tempral lobe lesions in man. *Neuropsychologia, 20*, 249–262.

[98] Shallice, T. (1982). Specific impairments of planning. *Philosophical transactions of Royal Society of London, 13*(298), 199–209.

[99] Milner, B. (1963). Effects of different brain lesions on card sorting. *Archives of Neurology, 9*, 90–100.

[100] Maj, M., Satz, P., Janssen, R., Zaudig, M., Startace, F., D'Elia, L. F., et al. (1994). WHO Neuropsychiatric AIDS study, cross sectional phase II: Neuropsychological and neurological fndings. *Archives of General Psychiatry, 51*, 51–61.

[101] Meyers, J., & Meyers, K. (1995). *Rey complex figure and recognition trial: Professional manual.* Florida: Psychological Assessment Resources.

[102] Thara, R., Padmavathi, R., Kumar, S., & Srinivasan, L. (1998). Burden assessment schedule: An instrument to assess burden in caregivers of chronic mentally ill. *Indian Journal of Psychiatry, 40*, 21–29.

[103] Eack, S. M., Greenwald, D. P., Hogarty, S. S., Cooley, S. J., DiBarry, A. L., Montrose, D. M., et al. (2009). Cognitive enhancement therapy for early-course schizophrenia: Effects of a two-year randomized controlled trial. *Psychiatric Services, 60*(11), 1468–1476.

[104] Ueland, T., & Rund, B. R. (2005). Cognitive remediation for adolescents with early onset psychosis: A 1-year follow-up study. *Acta Psychiatrica Scandinavica, 111*(3), 193–201.

[105] Gopal, Y. V., & Hannele, V. (2005). First-episode schizophrenia: Review of cognitive deficits and remediation. *Advances in Psychiatric Treatment, 11*, 38–44.

[106] Mueser, K. T. (2000). Cognitive functioning, social adjustment and long-term outcome in schizophrenia. In P. D. H. Tonmoy Sharma (Ed.), *Cognition in schizophrenia (pp. 157–177).* New York: Oxford University Press.

[107] Leff, J. (1994). Working with the families of schizophrenic patients. *The British Journal of Psychiatry, 164*(Suppl, 23), 71–76.

[108] Cassidy, E., Hill, S., & O'Callaghan, E. (2001). Efficacy of a psychoeducational intervention in improving relatives' knowledge about schizophrenia and reducing rehospitalisation. *European Psychiatry, 16*, 446–450.

[109] Barrowclough, C., Tarrier, N., Watts, S., Vaughn, C., Bamrah, J. S., & Freeman, H. L. (1987). Assessing the functional value of relatives' knowledge about schizophrenia: A preliminary report. *The British Journal of Psychiatry, 151*, 1–8.

[110] WHO, (2012). Mental Health-Schizophrenia, <http://www.who.int/mental_health/management/schizophrenia/en/>. World Health Organization.

[111] Rao, S. L. (2004). Cognitive dysfunction and cognitive remediation in schizophrenia. In Nizamie MKMnSH (Ed.), *Current Developments in Schizophrenia (pp. 304–339).* New Delhi: Allied Publishers Pvt. Ltd.

[112] Wagner, B. R. (1968). The training of attending and abstracting responses in chronic schizophrenics. *Journal of Experimental Research in Personality, 3*, 77–88.

[113] Meichenbaum, D., & Cameron, R. (1973). Training schizophrenics to talk to themselves: a means of developing attention controls. *Behavior Therapy, 4*, 515–534.

[114] Endicott, J., Spitzer, R. L., Fleiss, J. L., & Cohen, J. (1976). The global assessment scale. A procedure for measuring overall severity of psychiatric disturbance. *Arch Gen Psychiatry, 33*(6), 766–771.

[115] Goldberg, D. P., & Hillier, V. F. (1979). A scaled version of the general health questionnaire. *Psychol Med, 9*(1), 139–145.

[116] Noh, S., & Avison, W. R. (1987). Spouses of discharged psychiatric patients: factors associated with their experience of burden. *Journal of Marriage and Family, 50*(2), 377–389.

[117] Oldridge, M. L., & Hughes, I. C. (1992). Psychological well-being in families with a member suffering from schizophrenia. An investigation into long-standing problems. *Br J Psychiatry, 161*, 249–251.

[118] Hatfield, A., & Lefley, H. P. (2000). Helping elderly caregivers plan for the future care of a relative with mental illness. *Psychiatric Rehabilitation Journal, 24*, 103–107.

[119] Gidron, B. (1991). Stress and coping among Israeli parents of the mentally Ill. *International Social Work Journal, 34*(2), 159–170.

# 8 Neuropsychological Intervention for Specific Learning Disorder: An Innovative Approach

*A. Sadasivan*

Samvidh Psychological Services, Bangalore, Karnataka, India

Academic difficulties are common in school-going children. A severe difficulty in reading, writing, spelling, and calculation interferes with success in an academic setting among both children and adults. This difficulty, which affects academic performance despite adequate opportunities to learn, is referred to as specific learning disorder (SLD). The prevalence of SLD is reported all over the world, across different languages and education systems. It is estimated that in the United States alone about 20% of the school-going population has learning needs of one kind or another [1–3]. Conservative estimates with stringent diagnostic criteria report prevalence rates to be around 6–12.5% of the school-going population [4–6]. However, less conservative estimates place the prevalence at 20% of the school-going population.

Since the discovery of the disorder, researchers have struggled to arrive at a consensus regarding the terminology and definition of the disorder. Studies often vary in the way they define the problem. Traditional definitions assert that SLD exists when there is a significant discrepancy between a child's cognitive ability and achievement in reading, mathematics, or written expression [1]. In recent years, significant changes have occurred in the diagnostic criteria used for determining a SLD. Researchers argue that the earlier understanding of SLD on the basis of a discrepancy between achievement and ability has its limitations. Some researchers have argued against the discrepancy model as it places emphasis on average to above-average intellectual functioning. The most widely accepted definition of SLD considers it as a difficulty in reading, writing, calculation, and spelling despite adequate instruction and an opportunity to learn. In recent years, another model has been proposed, in which categorization of a child's SLD is based on a multitiered process involving, ideally, early identification and intervention, and review of response to intervention (RTI) [1].

One of the reasons for this discrepancy could be the heterogeneity of the representative population. The three primary SLDs are disorder of reading, mathematics, and written expression. A fourth learning disorder, not otherwise specified (LD-NOS), serves as a grouping for patterns of learning difficulty that are not

Neuropsychological Rehabilitation-Principles and Applications.
DOI: http://dx.doi.org/10.1016/B978-0-12-416046-0.00008-0

academic subject-specific (i.e., nonverbal learning disorder is characterized as LD-NOS). Children could present with one or more difficulties within the gamut of SLDs. In addition, they may have comorbid conditions such as language disorders, attention deficit hyperactivity disorder (ADHD), conduct disorder, and/or motor coordination disorder. In addition, about 65% of children with SLD are at risk for developing emotional and social difficulties which could further interfere with their day-to-day functioning. This contributes to the heterogeneity of the problem, thus making it difficult to establish a definition that can encompass various aspects of the difficulties. Understanding of children and adults with SLD solely on the basis of the DSM-IV-TR criteria thus might not be enough, especially if specific intervention is required.

Larkin and Ellis [7] reported some basic skills that are lacking in children with SLD. According to them, children with LD may:

1. lack basic skills required to meet academic demands,
2. fail to use adequate problem-solving strategies despite knowing them,
3. do not have or fail to use effective learning strategies,
4. have difficulty in learning new concepts at higher levels of complexity, and
5. fail to make gains with new/advanced inputs.

Three models have been described by Stassi and Tall [1] to understand SLD: the discrepancy model, the intraindividual differences model, and the RTI model. These models highlight the difference between the viewpoint of a special educator versus a neuropsychologist. Following is a brief description of the three models:

1. *Discrepancy Model:* According to the discrepancy model, any child known to have SLD is assessed for language proficiency, language expression, reading fluency, reading comprehension, written expression, mathematical calculation, and mathematical problem solving. Children who fall two standard deviations below normal in one or more of these tests are identified and referred to special education services and would be considered for receiving special accommodations under the respective education acts/departments. Current assessment and diagnostic practices in India use this model to identify and diagnose SLD in children [8,9].
2. *Intraindividual Differences Model:* This model holds that the academic discrepancy model is not sufficient to understand the entire gamut of difficulties a child faces. Instead it would be beneficial to assess the child on a range of neuropsychological tests to help identify both strengths and weaknesses. This would help develop a remedial program appropriate to the child's needs. The focus is on the differences within a child rather than between children. In recent years neuropsychologists have argued in favor of this model. They argue that neuropsychological deficits and strengths are found within this population. Thus, any assessment and remedial program would have to target deficits and utilize strengths in order to address the unique needs of each individual.
3. *Problem-Solving Model:* The third model is known as the problem-solving model or the RTI model. The proponents of this model do not believe that standardized tests are the only way to identify individuals with learning disorders. Instead, they propose that through behavioral observations and rating scales it would be possible to identify children with remedial needs earlier on. This model suits those individuals who have behavioral and/or emotional needs secondary to their learning difficulties. Psychologists understand that children with learning disorder present with social and emotional difficulties and that the

population is heterogeneous in its presentation [2,4,5]. Without the use of standardized tests it would be difficult to assess the presence and extent of the deficits. As this model does not insist on standardized assessment tools, it has been criticized as nonempirical [1].

The discrepancies between the various models and the large number of diagnostic criteria available in the literature is evidence of the heterogeneity present in SLD. Thus a wide range of tests that would cover all aspects of the disorder would be required to arrive at an understanding of the deficits that a child with SLD might have. Neuropsychological models of SLD have come a long way in dealing with the entire gamut of deficits seen in SLD. With the advent of neuroimaging techniques such as functional magnetic resonance imaging, single photon emission tomography, and diffusion tensor imaging, neuropsychologists have been able to identify anatomical regions responsible for carrying out functions such as reading, spelling, writing, and calculation. Based on these observations, theories have been formulated to help understand the disorders, develop assessment batteries, and design intervention techniques. Following is a brief description of the various forms of SLD and the neuroanatomical regions assumed to be involved in each of the deficits.

## Specific Reading Disorder

Reading is a complex act that involves several processes occurring simultaneously and smoothly [10]. While acquisition of spoken language is innate, reading has to be taught. Through instruction and adequate exposure, individuals become proficient readers [4]. There exists a difference between beginning (young) readers and skilled (older) readers in that they are known to employ different strategies to read and comprehend text. Beginning readers use an effortful process that involves decoding of individual sounds and words in order to access a word's meaning. Skilled readers can access a word's meaning more quickly because they have had prior experience reading and comprehending the word, which allows them to visually recognize a word based on both phonological and orthographic information. Reading for the skilled readers becomes "automatic"; able readers do not need to break a word into its individual sounds in order to read it [6,11,12]. A young/novice reader would start decoding the word using phonological principles. As the reader gains proficiency, speed and fluency of reading develop, allowing the reader to focus on reading quickly to derive meaning from the text. Normal development of the reading process allows a young/new reader to progress from one stage to another with exposure to text. However, with specific reading disorder this process is interrupted, and despite repeated exposure to text, some children find it difficult to progress from one stage to another, and therefore find it difficult to read words and/or text. Specific reading disorder is known to affect 5–15% of the school-going population [2,3,11]. The prevalence rates are influenced by several factors such as presence of associated comorbidities, the language used for reading, the presence of family history, and the presence of pressures within the education system. There are three popular theories that seek to explain the presence of reading disorder in children and adults: the phonological awareness deficit theory [5,6,11], the magnocellular theory [13–17], and the cerebellar theory [18–21].

Despite several criticisms, the most popular theory, which has stood the test of time, remains the phonological awareness deficit theory. According to this theory, reading involves several subcomponents such as phonological processing (required for the decoding of new and unfamiliar words), fluency and speed of reading, and reading comprehension. Each of these subcomponents requires specific neuro-anatomical regions to carry out the smooth functioning of the process of reading. Phonological processing and awareness require intact functioning of the left supra-marginal gyrus, left angular gyrus, perisylvian temporal lobes, larger right planum temporal, and left frontal regions [3,5]; reading speed and fluency require the intact functioning of dorsolateral prefrontal cortex, thalamus, magnocellular layers, and cerebellum [11,14]. Reading comprehension involves the superior temporal lobes, fusiform gyrus, and widespread frontal activity [1,11].

## Phonological Awareness in the Indian Context

Appreciation of the relationship between phonological awareness and early reading has its origin in the English-speaking nations. However, this awareness and under-standing spread to both European nations and other non-English-speaking nations. Although the sequence of phonological awareness development is similar across lan-guages, the subsyllabic units of which children become aware differ from one lan-guage to the next [22,23]. Researchers generally agree that the relationship between phonological awareness and the ability to read words holds for languages such as Spanish, German, English, and French, but not for nonalphabetic scripts [23]. Harris and Hatano [24] and Gowswami [22] agree that more cross-cultural research would be required before firm conclusions could be drawn, a claim that remains relevant today.

Eastern scripts, such as those of China, Japan, and India, do not support a strong relationship between phonological awareness and early reading skills [23]. Prakash et al. [25], Prakash and Rekha [26], and Prema and Karanth [27] have together estab-lished that phonological awareness is neither as evident nor as crucial to successful reading in Indian writing systems. The researchers found that children learning to read alphasyllabaries and adults who learned only one Indian language (Kannada or Hindi) performed well in rhyme recognition and syllable deletion tasks but did not perform well on segmentation tasks. In contrast, those who studied in both English and one Indian language (Kannada or Hindi) were able to carry out the phoneme segmentation tasks. Prakash and Rekha [26] found that children from Kannada medium schools showed a spurt in their performance on phoneme awareness tasks such as phoneme isolation and deletion after being introduced to English in the fourth grade. Karanth [23] concluded that the kinds of connections beginning readers make with phonology and orthography depend on the orthography of the language being learned.

Sharma (2000, unpublished dissertation) investigated the language skills of 23 Hindi-speaking children (7–15 years old) with reading disorder. None of the chil-dren was known to have oral language deficits. All were assessed on the Hindi ver-sion of the Linguistic Profile Test [28] (Sharma, 1995, unpublished dissertation), which evaluates language at phonological, syntactic, and semantic levels. The study indicated that the children with reading disorder had a lower language age (below 6 years) than those without. The deficits of the older children were more pronounced, especially relative to the more complex aspects of language abilities. A similar finding was reported for 21 Malayalam-speaking children (6–15 years of age). (Malayalam is another Indian language.) All 21 children had greater language deficits than phonological deficits. The older children showed a higher incidence of deficits than did the younger children.

## Specific Mathematical Disorder

Also known as dyscalculia or developmental mathematical disorder, specific mathematical disorder is known to affect 2–6% of the school-going population [29]. The prevalence rates reported vary from study to study as there is poor consensus among researchers about the definition of this disorder. Several authors agree that understanding of the disorder is in its infancy compared to the understanding of reading disorder [29]. Causal factors are reported to be possibly genetic as dyscalculia is reported in several genetic disorders such as Turner's syndrome, fragile X syndrome, and velocardiofacial syndrome. In addition, factors such as premature birth and prenatal exposure to alcohol are said to affect mathematical abilities in children. ADHD and reading disorder are known to be comorbid disorders associated with dyscalculia.

Deficits in dyscalculia include difficulties in understanding the association between a number and the quantity it represents (e.g., the number 5 represents five stones/bags/coins); understanding aspects of counting and its use in addition and subtraction; remembering and recalling of arithmetic facts and verbal and visuospatial skills that are required for solving algebra and geometry. Not all children have difficulties in all these areas. Wilson et al. [29] cited subtypes of dyscalculia. These include:

1. The *procedural subtype* is characterized by difficulties in counting and using the procedures of counting in solving problems. Individuals are thought to exhibit deficits in executive functions.
2. The *semantic subtype* is characterized by deficits in retrieving arithmetic facts. This subtype presents with verbal memory deficits and is reported to have dyslexia as a comorbidity.
3. The *visuospatial subtype* is characterized by deficits in visuospatial functioning. This subtype, however, is reported to be associated more with acquired dyscalculia rather than with developmental dyscalculia by some authors.

Dyscalculia is a heterogeneous disorder with deficits in three cognitive abilities required for success in performing mathematical operations. These include semantic memory, procedural memory, and visuospatial skills. Anatomical regions that are required for intact functioning include the bilateral intraparietal sulcus [29,30]. In addition, associated functions draw upon other regions of the brain to facilitate solving mathematical problems. The phonological loop, situated in the temporal regions, is required for retrieval of facts and for understanding word problems. Divided and sustained attention and the ability to manipulate and hold facts while calculating requires the frontal lobes and the anterior cingulated regions. Visual, spatial, and kinesthetic information, comparing of quantities, estimating size, and computation require the intact functioning of the bilateral parietal regions.

Though recent years have thrown light upon the neuroanatomical regions involved in or required for mathematical functioning, little is known regarding the remedial/ intervention strategies required to help children and adults overcome this disorder.

## Disorders of Written Expression

Also known as dysgraphia, disorder of written expression refers to inability of the child to express his/her ideas and thoughts through words in written format. The skill of writing is a complex activity involving many components, such as an ability to spell words correctly, and to organize thoughts and present them in a coherent and logical fashion such that the reader is able to understand the ideas of the writer. A disorder of writing can present with one or more deficits in the skills mentioned above. The prevalence of the disorder is difficult to estimate. The disorder is often found in conjunction with dyslexia or dyscalculia, and thus estimates are difficult as it is rare to find a child with dysgraphia alone. In addition, discrepancies in defining the disorder and the variance in policies regarding acceptable written expressions within the school curriculum have further made estimating prevalence of dysgraphia difficult. However, some studies place prevalence at 6% of the school-going population [1,29].

According to Stassi and Tall [1], the development of written expression consists of a set of neurocognitive components including understanding language and its rules, executive functions of organizing thought, self-monitoring and memory of facts, spelling ability, and rules of grammar, in addition to visuomotor and graphomotor components of writing. These cognitive abilities draw heavily on the functioning of the frontal and temporal lobes, i.e., areas involved in controlling executive functions, verbal memory, and language.

From the descriptions of the different kinds of learning disorders and their subtypes, it is evident SLD is not a simple condition involving one or a few neurocognitive abilities. Instead it refers to a range of difficulties, and no two children with learning difficulties are known to be alike in the range of difficulties they present with or in their responses to intervention. In short, the population is very heterogeneous, making the process of developing remedial programs a challenging task [2,8,28]. Prior to beginning a remedial program a detailed assessment would help in obtaining a profile of the child's strengths and weaknesses. The usual procedure is to assess the child's intellectual functions using a range of tests. The Wechsler's Intelligence Scale (WISC) is the preferred tool as it offers the unique advantage of assessing both verbal and performance tests along with a global IQ score. However, several researchers feel that assessment of intellectual functioning is not necessary for the diagnosis of SLD [31]. Tests of academic abilities such as reading, spelling, writing, and mathematical abilities are required for a diagnosis. Children falling two standard deviations below the expected score are considered to have SLD. Recent studies have established neurocognitive deficits in this population and thus the need for a neuropsychological evaluation in addition to intelligence and academic abilities is becoming increasingly popular [2]. Thus it would be useful to assess attention, working memory, mental flexibility, planning, and organization in addition to visual and verbal functions in this population. However, frequent usage of tests increases type I errors, and hence a careful balance in the choice and number of tests to evaluate the child's profile is advised [1]. The assessment provides a profile of both the child's strengths and weaknesses. This is helpful is considering the specific remedial strategies for a given child.

Several remedial strategies and programs have been described as being useful in SLD. Most of the evidence-based remedial programs quoted in the literature have been developed to help improve reading disorder. However, very few researchers (if any) have considered developing remedial programs for writing and mathematical disorders. Fewer still have provided guidelines for remedial strategies for children having more than one learning disorder. Clinicians working with this population are often faced with the challenge of working with children with multiple learning difficulties and with comorbid clinical conditions. In addition, it is now known that children with SLD also have neurocognitive deficits. Hence, considering a program such as phonological awareness (which is proved to be beneficial for reading disorder alone) might not suit the needs of all children or might not be an answer to all the difficulties a given child is facing. Hence, it is proposed that a broad-based remedial program, such as a neuropsychological remedial program, would address all the difficulties that a child with SLD might face.

## Specific Learning Disorder in the Indian Context

India is the seventh largest country in the world in terms of geographical area and has a population of about 1.2 billion people. People from different states in India speak different languages. There are 22 official languages in India, with each state having its own official language. In addition to these are the national language (Hindi) and English, both are important languages that the majority of Indian people use for communication [32].

India's education system reflects the influence of language on the learning process. The medium of instruction in the school can be English or the regional language. Children studying in schools learn all subjects in the language chosen as the medium of instruction. They also learn one or two languages other than the medium of instruction as core subjects in their curriculum. Assessment of language and its processes, therefore, is difficult to develop and standardize.

## The School System in India

Most Indians are exposed to and can speak more than one language. English is not the language primarily spoken in all homes, which means that many children are not formally exposed to it until they enter school. Being exposed to more than one language during the formative years influences the development of reading in Indian children. Researchers working in the field of language development and typical development of reading are therefore sensitive to the influence of multiple languages in these children.

In addition to the influence of the language used, other variations are seen in India's school system [8]. Urban and rural schools fall under the state syllabus of education or the central syllabus of education. The state syllabus is followed to a large extent in the rural regions and often has the regional language as the medium of instruction. In urban settings, other streams of education run alongside the state syllabus. These include the Indian Certificate of Secondary Education (ICSE) and the Central Board of Secondary Education (CBSE), both of which come under the central syllabus and use English as their medium of instruction. The state syllabus is a relatively easier program of study than the central system and is the one most often adopted by schools run by a state government. The more difficult central syllabus is mostly adopted by privately or centrally funded schools [8]. Children of low socio-economic status and from rural regions most often go to government-run schools. Most urban children attend aided or private schools that follow the state, ICSE, or CBSE syllabus.

## Prevalence of Learning Disorder in India

Reading represents the means by which much of the information presented in school is learned and is often implicated in poor academic performance and, from there, school failure [32]. Reasons for failure include, among others, the presence of learning disorders. About 80% of children diagnosed with learning disorder have specific reading disorder [23].

Epidemiological studies in India in the field of learning disorders—and specifically in reading disorder—have gained importance only during the last decade [33,34]. Suresh and Sebastain [35] found a high prevalence of specific reading disorder in rural areas. Yadav and Agarwal [36] estimate the prevalence of the disorder at 2.25%, with higher prevalence for boys than girls. However, the difficulty of estimating the exact prevalence in India is compounded by several factors, such as bilingualism/multilingualism, poor awareness among teachers, large numbers of children per class, and unavailability of adequate tools to evaluate children with reading disorder [23,36].

In their study, Tripathi and Kar [37] evaluated the prevalence rates of learning disorders in schools in and around Allahabad, a city in the northern part of India. They found a high prevalence of reading-related problems in Classes 2–5, with the prevalence diminishing across Classes 6–8. The authors found that specific problems in reading, such as letter-sound omissions, substitution, reversals, difficulties in fluency, and reading the same line again, were high across all classes. They also found writing difficulties across all class levels. Tripathi and Kar [37] concluded that the high prevalence of writing difficulties could be explained by the high emphasis on writing skills in the school curriculum.

Current understanding of learning disorder in India depends on literature from other English-speaking countries. Western assessment practices, instructional materials and intervention methods are strongly influential [38]. Most tests and screening tools used to identify children with SLD are either tools developed in the West or adaptations to suit Indian conditions. Some indigenous tools such as the NIMHANS SLD Index are available for use in English. Tools sensitive to the local languages, such as the Reading Acquisition Profile in Kannada, developed by Prema (1998, Unpublished doctoral dissertation), are also in use. Shankaranarayana [39] used letter identification, word recognition, and reading texts along with Western tests such as rhyming, Torgesen elision, rapid automatized naming, rapid alternating stimulus, short-term memory for digits, conservation, handedness, and vocabulary. She found that the best predictors of reading ability for the Indian sample were speed of naming letters, vocabulary, and phonological awareness.

Rozario [40] prepared an informal reading inventory by carefully selecting graded reading passages and identifying specific reading errors. He used a similar procedure for assessing spelling and writing disorders. Rozario [40] recommended that each individual's strengths and weaknesses be identified in order to develop a highly individualized profile of the individual's cognitive and personality styles [38].

## Interventions for Specific Learning Disorder in India

In India, when children with specific reading disorder are identified, depending on the severity of the reading difficulty, they attend either a special school or a regular school while attending remedial sessions for a few hours a day. Several remedial centers use individual educational programs based on the assessment profile of the child. Only a few educational and clinical psychologists develop and/or use remedial programs. Carefully controlled intervention studies for specific reading disorder for children in India are scarce, and their approaches and outcomes vary. This section presents three such studies.

Rozario [40] described a remedial training program consisting of training on phonics, sight word reading, and language skills. Srikanth and Karanth [41] used a remedial program based on the Aston Teaching Program. With both these studies, cases were assessed and remedial work was done that kept in mind individual error patterns and areas of difficulty. The remediation focused on auditory visual channel, specific spelling rules and cues, comprehension skills, oral expression, and visuomotor perceptual aspects. The authors concluded that a complete remedial program should aim at both reading and spoken language proficiency.

Padegar and Sarnath [42] assessed three children in the age range of 7–11 years who had been referred to the Maharashtra Dyslexia Association resource center for remediation of severe reading disorder. All three children had above-average intelligence. They were assessed on word attack and word identification subtests before and after intervention. The intervention program used was the Planning, Attention-Arousal, Simultaneous and Successive (PASS), Processing Reading Enhancement Program (PREP) [43]. This program for primary-school children aims to improve information-processing strategies, specifically the simultaneous and successive processing that underlies reading, without direct teaching of phonological skills such as phoneme blending and segmentation. The authors compared the assessment profile of these three children with three other children with specific reading disorder who received regular remedial training consisting of training on phonics, sight word reading, and a whole language approach. Both interventions were administered in 24 sessions. The control group received only remedial training while the PREP group received PREP as well as remedial training once a week. Results showed improvements for both groups, but the PREP group showed an increase in their word identification and word-attack skills after intervention.

Special remedial centers around the country use a combination of methods drawing primarily from multimodal stimulation strategies. Worksheets are prepared to teach concepts, and these worksheets approach the concept from various angles, allowing the child ample opportunity to learn using more than one modality. Verbal, visual, kinesthetic, and tactile modalities are explored in addition to the traditional auditory and verbal methods of approaching a concept. Under this strategy, each component of learning is treated independently, and strategies are taught in order to bring about an improvement in specific skills. For example, if the child has difficulty in reading, the strategies to improve reading are taught using worksheets. Short- and long-term goals are set based on the child's basal levels, and an attempt is made to consider lessons from the curriculum of the child so that he/she is able to function on a par with the other children in the class.

In recent years, schools have been known to set up what are referred to as resource rooms, where interventions based on principles of special education are offered to the child during school hours. This is to reduce the burden on parents and to allow the child to remain in mainstream education while still obtaining the benefits of intervention. In the resource rooms, special educators and psychologists assess the child referred by the class teacher. Based on the findings of the assessment, an individualized educational plan is drawn for the child. This plan is communicated to the teacher, who is then able to work with the child. In addition, the child is sent to the resource room for further help with enhancing associated difficulties such as attention, visuospatial skills, and memory. Following is a brief description of some of the strategies commonly used by special educators:

*Reading and spelling*: Reading is a complex skill requiring knowledge of word/letter sound association. Following are some tips and strategies used to enhance reading.

1. Teaching the child specific sounds of the letters. Separation of vowels from consonants is essential as consonant sounds tend to be more stable than vowel sounds. After the child is familiar with consonant sounds, then short-vowel sounds and then long-vowel sounds are introduced in order to facilitate the understanding of how vowel sounds affect the reading and spelling of words.
2. Lists of monosyllabic words (usually monosyllables are used), for example, the Dolch lists. The child is presented repeatedly with these words, starting from simple and moving to more complex words. These are words that frequently appear in text, such as "it," "an," "was," "saw," "them," and "their." Words are presented on independent cards, and the child is encouraged to rapidly read the word. As the child reaches about 80% accuracy at a given level, the next level is approached.
3. Once a child has gained knowledge of phonemes, this knowledge is transferred to the syllable level. The child is introduced to multisyllable (two or more syllables) words and is taught to split the word into its syllables and then read/spell it.

**4.** From word level the child is encouraged to read at the sentence level using the aforementioned strategies and then reading with more text.

**5.** Spelling rules and exceptions to spelling rules are taught where required to help children spell both regular and irregular words with ease.

**6.** Once the child has achieved these stages, he/she is encouraged to read text in a graded manner. His/her comprehension of the text is monitored and strategies to revise and question the meaning within the text are explored.

*Writing*: Writing consists of two aspects: first, the motor component, where the formation of the letter, the neatness and speed of writing, and the grip of the pencil/pen are assessed. The second aspect refers to the content. In younger children, the first aspect is of primary concern while as the child grows older the focus shifts from handwriting to the content of what is written. Following are some strategies used to help children write better:

**1.** Children are encouraged to actively use the reading/spelling strategies learned while they attempt to write words/sentences/paragraphs.

**2.** Rules of grammar such as use of tenses, parts of speech, relationships between words, and the meaning of words based on context are taken up one by one. Each time the child writes, he/she is encouraged to use this knowledge and correct his/her written expression.

**3.** After he/she has written a piece, the child is encouraged to read and reread the text to monitor his/her own errors. Error monitoring is taught by allowing the child to identify errors in other texts and then gradually transfer this skill to his/her own writing.

**4.** When the child has to write a passage, he/she is encouraged to consider all the various aspects of the topic, prepare a plan on how he/she is going to present the ideas, and draw a map of what should come where and when. Once this exercise is fulfilled, the child is asked to write an essay.

*Mathematics*: Mathematics consists of several aspects, such as arithmetic, algebra, and geometry. As there are several related yet different concepts, intervention strategies for each of these are taken up independently. The child is initially allowed to understand the concept by working at the concept using concrete examples. From there, abstract examples are worked out at a later stage.

For example, when the child has to understand the concept of multiplication he/she is made to count in twos (for the two times table) or fives (for the five times table). Figure 8.1 shows how a child is taught the concept of multiplication. A child is shown pictures of two objects each. This way the child learns that two times two means two leaves two times is equal to four. The child is also taught, using the same visual aid, that multiplication is actually long addition.

The next step is to encourage the child to use lines instead of pictures to count, then directly add, and finally learn the table through rote. The same method can be used to teach fractions and decimals, percentages, etc.

The strategies discussed above are used for difficulty in a specific domain noticed in the child. However, as we are aware, children with SLD present with difficulties in more than one area. Hence, using the strategies mentioned increases the load on a child's memory as he/she has to remember several strategies and use them appropriately. Considering only one or two domains at a time might result in partial remediation. Hence, a more comprehensive program is required in order to address several

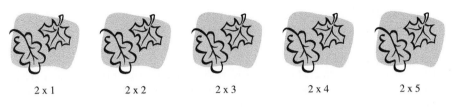

| 2 x 1 | 2 x 2 | 2 x 3 | 2 x 4 | 2 x 5 |

**Figure 8.1** Pictorial representation of multiples of two.

difficulties simultaneously. In addition, cognitive difficulties such as working memory or attention difficulties might interfere with the progress the child makes in the intervention program. Hence, a more broad-based intervention program would be time- and cost-effective.

## Issues Pertinent to the Indian Context

The review of children with specific reading disorder in the Indian context highlights several important issues. First, the education system and sociocultural differences pose a challenge to professionals working in the field. Second, the influence of many languages in the education system creates particular difficulty not only for children with specific reading disorder but also for those interested in assessing and remediating the disorder. Third, because Indian languages differ in structure from English, inferences drawn from Western populations may not be readily applicable to the Indian population. Finally, the use of Western tools of assessment and remedial training may not be effective for all groups of children with reading disorder across the country. While certain tools and remedial procedures might be relevant for children from English-medium schools, their relevance for the vernacular medium of schools is questionable.

Intervention for specific reading disorder poses another challenge in that intervention programs used effectively with English-speaking children may not be suitable for multilingual Indian children. In addition, the demands that the school places on children in India may be very different from the demands placed on children in other countries. Therefore, if an intervention program is to be effective in the Indian system, it must consider the demands placed by the education system on the child and the influences of his/her environment. In short, a program found to be effective in another country will not necessarily yield the same result in India.

Research has consistently pointed to the presence of neurocognitive deficits in children with learning disorder. Multiple anatomical regions are required to display intact functioning in order for a child to carry out the functions of reading, writing, spelling, or calculation. Therefore, a program that focuses on one or a few cognitions or abilities would only result in partial remediation. An effective remedial program would have to consider a heterogeneous population with multiple deficits and target multiple anatomical regions. A neuropsychological remedial program that focuses on several cognitions such as enhancing attention, executive functions, and memory (both verbal and visuospatial) would be able to address the needs of children with more than one learning disorder. In addition, in a country like India, a comprehensive program would be required to help the child cope with the demands of the academic system.

Sadasivan et al. [44] conducted a study to determine the effectiveness of two interventions (a phonologically based intervention and a neuropsychological-cognitive-based intervention) for reading disorder in a group of 20 children in the Indian education system. The phonologically based intervention has proven effective in meeting the needs of Australian and New Zealand monolingual English-speaking children [45], and its effectiveness in another educational environmental context was compared with the neuropsychological intervention program specifically developed for this study. The study found that both the remedial programs showed improvement in reading accuracy. The phonological group showed significant changes in verbal fluency, visual scanning and attention, word reading, verbal memory, immediate visual memory, and visuoconstruction abilities.

Phonological measures that showed significant increase in RTI in this group included nonword reading, phoneme detection, phoneme segmentation, phoneme deletion, and tracking of syllable sound changes via use of colored blocks and letter tiles. The neuropsychological group showed significant changes in neuropsychological functions such as verbal fluency, word reading and interference control, verbal learning, immediate visual memory, and visuoconstruction ability. The neuropsychological group also improved significantly on phonological awareness measures such as syllable identification, spoken and visual rhyme, spoonerism, phoneme detection, phoneme deletion, and tracking of syllable sound changes via use of colored blocks. Both groups maintained the gains they had made 3 months after the program was terminated. The study advanced understanding of the relevance of a broad-based remedial program within the context of the Indian education system. It also established that the two remedial programs helped improve reading abilities equally. However, the interventions differentially affected neuropsychological and phonological awareness functioning in the participants.

Following is a description of a child who showed improvement in phonological, neuropsychological, behavioral, and academic domains after receiving a brief neuropsychological intervention.

## Case Vignette

HK, an 11-year-old boy studying in Class 6, was referred by his teachers for assessment. HK was adopted when he was a few months old. HK's adoptive father was unable to provide information about HK's biological parents or why he was given up for adoption. At the time of evaluation, the parents reported both behavioral problems and academic difficulties. The academic difficulties identified were poor and sloppy handwriting, inability to complete notes on time, difficulty in remembering answers learned at home, poor spelling abilities, and poor comprehension of text matter. The parents also reported that HK could read quickly and with some ease if the words were familiar to him. However, he could understand little of what he read. He avoided reading passages with difficult words and said that he could not understand the text. His parents would then have to explain the text a few times before he could understand. HK also failed to remember much of what he learned at home. As a result of all these problems, HK's academic record showed a consistent drop in performance, a drop that had been particularly steep over the previous 3 years.

HK showed poor motivation to study and avoided any study time. His playtime often extended beyond the permissible limit, and he would end up having little time to finish his homework. His schoolwork remained incomplete, as his writing was slow and illegible. His books got misplaced, and he was reported to be careless with them. He was comfortable playing with children younger than himself, and his behavior was generally noticed to be inappropriate for his age. He did not learn from his mistakes and continued to display behavioral difficulties despite being punished for them.

The parents furthermore reported that HK was easily distracted but that his inattention was restricted to his study time. If he was engaged in an activity that interested him, he could sustain his attention until he had completed the task. He was also known to be a very kind and sensitive child, and would please his grandfather by showing affection and following religious traditions when required.

An assessment was carried out to identify the severity of his problems. The assessment revealed that HK was reading at Class 4 level (both accuracy and comprehension were intact at this level). Since HK was in Class 6 at the time of assessment, the reading assessment revealed that he was 2 years below his expected level of reading. Math skills were found to be age appropriate. His score on the Raven's Progressive Matrices (RPM) placed him in the average range of intellectual functioning. The diagnosis reached was that of specific learning difficulty with behavior problems.

HK received his neuropsychological intervention 2 days a week for 10 weeks (20 sessions) for a period of 3.6 months. HK was initially given letter cancellation, shading, and grain sorting. These tasks were used initially as attention tasks because of his being easily distracted. On the letter-cancellation task, HK was asked to cancel two letters wherever they appeared in the text provided. He was given 10 min to work on this activity. HK made several omissions and could not complete the task within the given time. His shading was clumsy and dark with excess pressure, and he was unable to follow the instructions given while shading (i.e., to reduce pressure, to make the shading even and light, and to restrict shading to within the given boundaries). As the intervention progressed, he was able to reduce pressure and shade within the drawn boundary. The number of errors he made in his letter-cancellation task were reduced, suggesting that he had probably gained adequate attentional control on the tasks after 20 sessions.

Tasks such as verbal fluency, temporal ordering, and frequency ordering were proposed to enhance HK's executive functions, such as mental search organization and planning and encoding of information. At first HK found verbal fluency a challenge, as he was not able to generate more than five to seven words in the 2 min allotted for each letter. He was given strategies on how to search for words beginning with a particular letter. For example, he was asked to think of the possible sound the letter would make and to use that as a cue to search for words. He was also asked to add other letter sounds (phonemes) to the target letter to see how many words he could identify. He was able to act on these instructions: his verbal fluency showed improvement, and toward the end of the intervention he was able to generate more than 20 words per letter in a span of 2 min. HK found temporal ordering the most difficult of all his tasks, as he could not make sentences with the disconnected words. During this activity, he was presented with a list of words divided into three segments. The number of words in each segment varied depending on the child's performance. For HK, the initial list consisted of six words divided into three segments of two words each. HK was presented with the first two words and asked to make one sentence using both words in the same sentence. He then had to visualize the sentence and hold onto the two words given. This procedure was repeated for the other two segments. Finally, he had to recall all six words in the list. In one session, three such lists were given. Once HK could recall at least five to six words on each list, the length of the list was increased to 9 (with three words per segment), 12 words (four words per segment), and 15 words (five words per segment).

The jump from a list of six words to nine was quick for HK. However, the jump from 9 to 12 words took him a long time, as he was unable to make sentences with different words. The themes/ideas he expressed in his sentences remained very similar. For example, for the words needle, pen, and table, he made this sentence: "The pen and needle were on the table." For the next set of words (rope, paper, and cycle), he said, "The paper and rope were on the cycle." He was given feedback on this repetition and asked to consider actively using the objects in his sentences, as that would enhance his ability to remember them.

As his performance across the three lists got better at using concrete and related words, he began to encounter the abstract or unrelated words in the lists, thus increasing the difficulty level for him. In addition, on the third list, HK was asked to make the sentence in his mind rather than speak it out. This meant that the extra auditory feedback he would get by repeating the sentence and the words was withdrawn. HK had to hold all the words without repeating them to the examiner several times, as in the other two trials. (This trial was named the neutral trial.) Thus, he was tested for recall of material that he organized in his mind without external cues. Forgetting was noticed initially on these trials, despite HK having 100% accurate recall on the other two lists of similar length and difficulty level. As the training progressed, he was able to remember all the words, even if all three trials were neutral lists. By the end of the 20 sessions, however, he reported being comfortable generating sentences using four words in a group.

Continuous phoneme tapping and mental math were used as working memory tasks. The former was hypothesized to be a passive working memory task that required HK to report whether the word presented contained a particular phoneme or not. HK had to tap the table to indicate the presence of the phoneme in the words. If he did not tap when the word had the target phoneme or if he tapped for a word that did not have the phoneme, it was counted as an error. Errors were 10 per trial initially, later reducing to 3.

When working on the mental mathematics task, HK initially found it very difficult to remember the previous number, and he required assistance for this. He took longer to complete the task and also had increased errors. By the end of the 20 sessions, he was able to hold onto the previous number, both rapidly and accurately. The target numbers were then made more difficult by including larger numbers (6–9) and dropping smaller numbers such as 1 and 2 for adding. Thus, accuracy, speed, and difficulty levels were changed to enhance active mental manipulations. HK made gains on all the treatment tasks and reached saturation levels so that the next difficulty level could be introduced.

In his report, HK said that he enjoyed all the tasks. He found the mental mathematics task very challenging, but said he wanted to get to the more difficult levels quickly. On the fluency task, he at first asked for specific letters so that he could easily get to a target of 20 words in 2 min. In later sessions, he asked for letters that he felt he needed more practice with. He showed keen interest in getting feedback on his performance and noted the difference between the present and the previous performance. In this way, he constantly challenged himself and showed good motivation to reach goals that were set on the basis of his previous performance.

After HK had completed his 20 sessions, conducted across 3.6 months, he was assessed in the week following the intervention program on neuropsychological and phonological awareness tests. Five months later, he was assessed on the neuropsychological tests and nonword reading, reading passages, and phoneme segmentation. The results of these two assessments are presented in Figures 8.2–8.5, along with the pretreatment assessment.

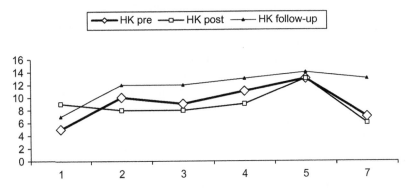

**Figure 8.2 HK's performance on verbal learning and memory measures.**
1 = number of words recalled on Trial 1 of Ray Auditory Verbal Learning Test (AVLT); 2 = number of words recalled on Trial 2 of AVLT; 3 = number of words recalled on Trial 3 of AVLT; 4 = number of words recalled on Trial 4 of AVLT; 5 = number of words recalled on Trial 5 of AVLT; 7 = number of words recalled after 20-min delay on AVLT.

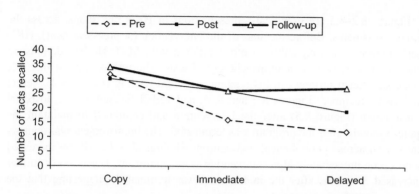

**Figure 8.3 HK's visual perception and visual memory across three assessments.** Copy: visual perception measured on complex figure test; Immediate: immediate visual memory measured on complex figure test; Delayed: delayed visual recall on complex figure test.

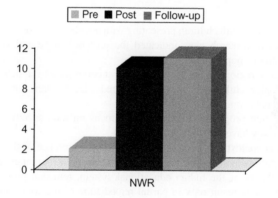

**Figure 8.4** HK's nonword reading performance across three assessments. NWR, nonword reading.

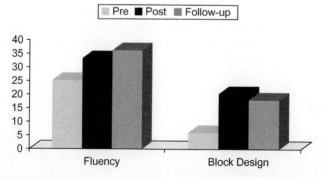

**Figure 8.5** HK's fluency and block design performance across three assessments.

Figures 8.2–8.5 are graphical representations of HK's raw scores across the three assessments. Before the start of the intervention (at preassessment), HK's performance was comparable to other children with SLD. He had deficits on phonological as well as neuropsychological tests. The results suggest that HK made significant progress in his reading, nonword reading (Figure 8.4), verbal and visual memory (Figures 8.2 and 8.3), and verbal fluency and visuospatial construction (Figure 8.5) after the intervention and continued to maintain the gains 3 months after the program was terminated. The improvement was consistently seen across phonological and neuropsychological tests. All the increased scores seen immediately after intervention were significant. These scores further increased 3 months after the intervention was terminated, suggesting that the improvement was maintained.

## Conclusion

- SLD is heterogeneous, with children presenting with a wide variety of signs and symptoms.
- Recent advances in research have indicated the presence of several cognitive domains found in deficit in this population.
- Specific anatomical regions carrying out specific functions have been delineated.
- Typically developing children have been compared with children with SLD in order to arrive at these conclusions.
- Specific intervention programs already existing focus only on specific deficit functions. These studies mostly have stemmed from the West.
- Within the Indian context few studies have explored the presence of the deficits and have established the presence of the disorder across different vernacular languages.
- Given the complexity of the Indian educational system, remedial programs focusing on specific functions may result only in partial remediation of the wide range of difficulties these children face.
- Hence, a need for a comprehensive program that can address a wide range of difficulties is required in order to facilitate mainstreaming of children within a more demanding education system.
- A neuropsychologically driven program that considers addressing the base cognitions across all domains is proposed to be more beneficial than compartmentalizing cognitive processes.
- The chapter proposes one such program that has brought about positive changes.
- More such studies are required to establish this in a larger sample.

## References

[1] Stassi, G. M., & Tall, L. G. (2010). Learning disorders in children and adolescents. In J. Donders, & S. J. Hunters (Eds.), *Principles and practice of lifespan developmental neuropsychology*. Cambridge: Cambridge University Press.
[2] Katzir, T. (2008). How research in the cognitive neuroscience sheds lights on subtypes of children with dyslexia: Implications for teachers [Electronic Version]. *Cortex*.

[3] Shaywitz, S. E., & Shaywitz, B. A. (2005). Dyslexia (specific reading disability). *Biological Psychiatry, 57*, 1301–1309.

[4] Shaywitz, S. E. (2003). Dyslexia. *The New England Journal of Medicine, 338*(5), 307–312.

[5] Ramus, F. (2003). Developmental dyslexia: Specific phonological deficit or general sensorimotor dysfunction. *Current Opinion in Neurobiology, 13*, 1–7.

[6] Habib, M. (2000). The neurological basis of developmental dyslexia: An overview and working hypothesis [review]. *Brain, 123*(12), 2373–2399.

[7] Larkin, M, & Ellis, E. (1998). In B. Y. L. Wong (Ed.), *Learning about learning disabilities* (pp. 557–577). New York: Academic Press.

[8] Kapur, M. (2008). In K. Thapa, G. Aalsvoort, M. Van Der, & J. Pandey (Eds.), *Perspectives on learning disabilities in India: Current practices and prospects* (pp. 80–96). New Delhi: Sage Publications.

[9] Kapur, M., Barnabas, I., Reddy, M. V., Rozario, J., & Hirisave, U. (Eds.), (2002). *Assessment of psychopathology checklist for children (DPCL)*. Bangalore, India: NIMHANS Publications.

[10] Price, C. J. (2000). The anatomy of language: Contributions from functional neuroimaging. *Journal of Anatomy, 197*, 335–359.

[11] Frackowiak, R. S. J., Friston, K. J., Frith, C. D., Dolan, R. J., Price, C. J., Zeki, S. et al. (Eds.), (2004). *Human Brain Function*. London: Elsevier Press.

[12] Geschwind, N., & Galaburda, A. M. (1985). Cerebral lateralization. Biological mechanisms, associations, and pathology: I. A hypothesis and a program for research. *Archives of Neurology, 5*(42), 428–459.

[13] Tallal, P. (1980). Auditory temporal perception, phonics, and reading disabilities in children. *Brain and Language, 9*, 182–198.

[14] Temple, E., Deutsch, G. K., Poldrack, R. A., Miller, S. L., Tallal, P., Merzenich, M. M., et al. (2003). Neural deficits in children with dyslexia ameliorated by behavioral remediation: Evidence from functional MRI. *Proceedings of the National Academy of Sciences of the United States of America, 100*(5), 2860–2865.

[15] Skottun, B. C. (2005). Magnocellular reading and dyslexia. *Vision Research, 45*(1), 133–134.

[16] John, S. (2001). The magnocellular theory of developmental dyslexia. *Dyslexia, 7*(1), 12–36.

[17] Stuart, G. W., McAnally, K. I., & Castles, A. (2001). Can contrast sensitivity functions in dyslexics be explained by inattention rather than a magnocellular deficit? *Australian Journal of Psychology, 53*, 46.

[18] Howard, J. H., Howard, D. V., Japikse, K. C., & Eden, G. F. (2006). Dyslexics are impaired on implicit higher-order sequence learning, but not on implicit spatial context learning. *Neuropsychologia, 44*, 1131–1144.

[19] Nicolson, R. I., & Fawcett, A. J. (1990). Automacity: A new framework for dyslexia research? *Cognition, 35*, 159–182.

[20] Nicolson, R. I., Fawcett, A. J., & Dean, P. (1995). Time estimation deficits in developmental dyslexia: Evidence of cerebellar involvement. *Proceedings of the Royal Society of London Series B—Biological Sciences, 259*, 43–47.

[21] Nicolson, R. I., Fawcett, A. J., & Dean, P. (2001). Dyslexia, development and the cerebellum. *Trends in Neuroscience, 24*, 515–516.

[22] Gowswami, U. (1999). The relationship between phonological awareness and orthographic representation in different orthography. In G. A. K. Thappa, M. Van Der, & J. Pandey (Eds.), *Perspectives on learning disabilities in India: Current practices and prospects* (pp. 80–96). New Delhi: Sage Publications.

[23] Karanth, P. (2008). Learning disability and language learning. In K. Thapa, G. Aalsvoort, M. Van Der, & J. Pandey (Eds.), *Perspectives on learning disabilities in India: Current practices and prospects* (pp. 80–96). New Delhi: Sage Publications.

[24] Harris, M., & Hatano, G. (1990). Learning to read and write: A cross-linguistic perspective. In G. A. K. Thappa, M. Van Der, & J. Pandey (Eds.), *Perspectives on learning disabilities in India: Current practices and prospects*. New Delhi: Sage Publications.

[25] Prakash, P., Rekha, R., Nigam, R., & Karanth, P. (1993). Phonological awareness, orthography and literacy. In R. Scholes (Ed.), *Literacy and language* (pp. 138–149). Mahwah, NJ: Lawerence Erlbaum Associates.

[26] Prakash, P., & Rekha, B. (1992). Phonological awareness and reading acquisition in Kannada. In A. K. Srivastava (Ed.), *Researches in child and adolescent psychology* (pp. 47–52). New Delhi: NCERT.

[27] Prema, K. S., & Karanth, P. (2003). Assessment of learning disability: Language based tests. In P. K. J. Rozario (Ed.), *Learning disabilities in India: Willing the mind to learn* (pp. 138–149). New Delhi: Sage Publications.

[28] Karanth, P. (1984). *Inter-relationship of linguistic deviance and social deviance.* Paper presented at the report on young scientists fellowship award. New Delhi: Indian Council of Social Science Research.

[29] Wilson, A. J., Revkin, S. K., Cohen, D., Cohen, L., & Dehaene, S. (2006). An open trial assessment of "The Number Race", an adaptive computer game for remediation of dyscalculia. *Behavioral and Brain Functions, 2*, 20.

[30] Geary, D. C., Hamson, C. O., & Hoard, M. K. (2000). Numerical and arithmetical cognition: A longitudinal study of process and concept deficits in children with learning disability. *Journal of Experimental Child Psychology, 77*, 236–263.

[31] Swanson, H. L., & Seigel, L. (2001). Learning disabilities as a working memory deficit. Issues in education. *Contributions from Educational Psychology, 7*, 1–48.

[32] Ministry of Information Broadcasting. (2009). *Manorama.* New Delhi.

[33] Thapa, K. (2008). Learning disabilities: Issues and concerns. In K. Thappa, G. Aalsvoort, M. Van Der, & J. Pandey (Eds.), *Perspectives on learning disabilities in India: Current practices and prospects* (pp. 23–47). New Delhi: Sage Publications.

[34] Karanth, P. (2003). Learning disabilities in India: Willing the mind to learn. In P. Karanth, & J. Rozario (Eds.), *Perspectives on learning disabilities in India: Current practices and prospects* (pp. 17–29). New Delhi: Sage Publications.

[35] Suresh, P. A., & Sebastain, S. (2003). Epidemiological and neurological aspects of learning disabilities. In P. Karanth, & J. Rozario (Eds.), *Learning disabilities in India: Willing the mind to learn* (pp. 30–43). New Delhi: Sage Publications.

[36] Yadav, D., & Agarwal, V. (2008). A base-line study of learning disabilities: Its prevalence, teacher awareness and classroom practices. In K. Thapa, G. Aalsvoort, M. Van Der, & J. Pandey (Eds.), *Perspectives on learning disabilities in India: Current practices and prospects* (pp. 221–238). New Delhi: Sage Publications.

[37] Tripathi, N., & Kar, B. R. (2008). Teachers' perception of learning-related problems in school-going children. In K. Thapa, G. Aalsvoort, M. Van Der, & J. Pandey (Eds.), *Perspectives on learning disabilities in India: Current practices and prospects* (pp. 200–220). New Delhi: Sage Publications.

[38] Verma, P. (2008). Learning disability: Challenges in diagnosis and assessment. In K. Thappa, G. M. V. Aalsvoort, & J. Pandey (Eds.), *Perspectives on learning disabilities in India: Current practices and prospects* (pp. 143–170). New Delhi: Sage Publications.

[39] Shankaranarayana, A. (2003). Cognitive profiles of children learning to read English as a second language. In P. Karanth, & J. Rozario (Eds.), *Learning disabilities in India: Willing the mind to learn* (pp. 77–90). New Delhi: Sage Publications.

[40] Rozario, J. (2003). Assessment of learning disabilities. In P. Karanth, & J. Rozario (Eds.), *Learning disabilities in India: Willing the mind to learn*. New Delhi: Sage Publications.

[41] Srikanth, N., & Karanth, P. (2003). Speech language pathologists and the remediation of reading disabilities. In P. Karanth, & J. Rozario (Eds.), *Learning disabilities in India: Willing the mind to learn*. New Delhi: Sage Publications.

[42] Padegar, S., & Sarnath, J. (2008). A theory-driven approach to the diagnosis and remediation of learning problems in children. In G. A. K. Thappa, M. Van Der, & J. Pandey (Eds.), *Perspectives on learning disabilities in India: Current practices and prospects* (pp. 238–254). New Delhi: Sage Publications.

[43] Dass, J. P., Naglieri, J. A., & Kirby, J. R. (1994). Assessment of cognitive processes: The PASS theory of intelligence. In K. Thapa, G. Aalsvoort, M. Van Der, & J. Pandey (Eds.), *Perspectives on learning disabilities in India: Current practices and prospects*. New Delhi: Sage Publications.

[44] Sadasivan, A., Gillon, G., & Rucklidge, J. (2009). The effects of phonological awareness intervention on neuropsychological functioning in children with reading disabilities. *New Zealand Speech and Language Therapy Journal, 64*, 12–25.

[45] Gillon, G., & Dodd, B. (1997). Enhancing the phonological processing skills of children with specific reading disability. *European Journal of Disorders of Communication, 32*, 67–90.

# 9 Neuropsychological Rehabilitation: Critical Analysis

## A. Nehra*, D. Sadana†, and J. Rajeswaran†

*Department of Clinical Neuropsychology, Neurosciences Center, All India Institute of Medical Sciences (AIIMS), New Delhi, India, †Department of Clinical Psychology, National Institute of Mental Health and Neurosciences (NIMHANS), Bangalore, Karnataka, India

*Criticism may not be agreeable, but it is necessary. It fulfills the same function as pain in the human body, by calling attention to an unhealthy state of things.*

**Winston Churchill**

To stipulate indicators of "an unhealthy state of things" in the burgeoning field of neuropsychology is a daunting challenge. It is difficult partly because each inadequacy manifests itself as an opportunity that can be capitalized on in the next moment. For a field to grow, it is imperative that it utilizes these opportunities and expands its horizons. Though the field of neuropsychological rehabilitation has its origins in World Wars I and II [1], it is still considered a budding science. It has been a long journey, and the field has achieved significant results; however, there still exists skepticism and ambiguity regarding its effectiveness, its empiricism, and future directions. In order to critically evaluate the progress of a field, it is essential to discern its developmental trajectory, current impediments, and challenges for the future.

Principles of cognitive rehabilitation were used with soldiers of the world wars who suffered brain injuries during combat and needed assistance with functional skills [1]. Rehabilitation centers were set up in all parts of the world, with emphasis on assessment of deficits, functional skills training, and maintenance of gains through long-term follow-up. The German government after World War I sent brain-injured warriors to "schools for soldiers" (rehabilitation centers) to ameliorate their cognitive deficits. In Europe, developed rehabilitation techniques, referring to them as "nervous and mental re-education," while in the former Soviet Union after World War II, Luria [36, 37] developed a variety of techniques by locating specific functions to specific brain regions [1]. Prigatano et al. [2], in a review of the historical development of cognitive rehabilitation, emphasize the remarkable contributions of Zangwill [38], who proposed the principles of restoration, substitution, and compensation [39], who proposed a functions-based holistic approach to rehabilitation; and Luria, who used localization theory in efforts to improve impaired brain functions. Many of the principles and techniques used today are derived from the works of these

Neuropsychological Rehabilitation-Principles and Applications.
DOI: http://dx.doi.org/10.1016/B978-0-12-416046-0.00009-2

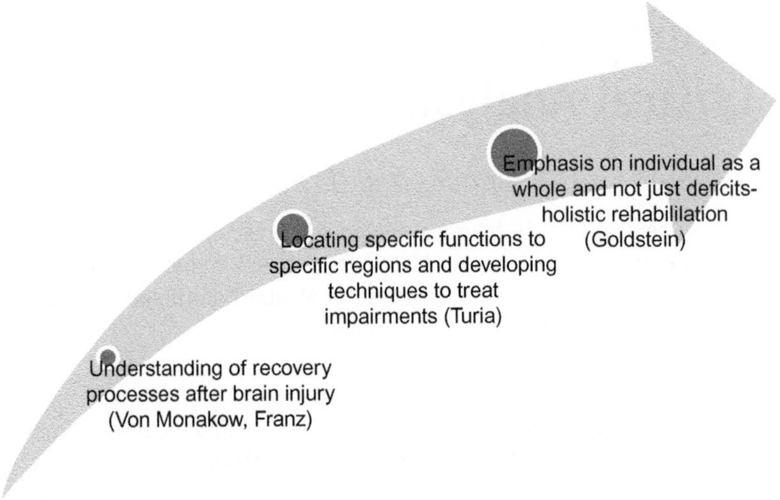

**Figure 9.1** Three landmark contributions in cognitive rehabilitation.

eminent clinicians (Figure 9.1). Prigatano [3], in his chapter on history of cognitive rehabilitation, referred to the works of these clinicians as "three great traditions that influence current practices."

During the 1970s and 1980s, the field of rehabilitation progressed with developments in cognitive psychology. As the processes of attention, perception, learning, and memory became better understood, the techniques to treat cognitive impairments became more refined. These developments fueled an increase in research and publications in the field, emphasizing the need and scope of rehabilitation [4–6]. Newcombe [7], in her review, describes cognitive rehabilitation as emerging from an amalgamation of experimental psychology, cognitive psychology, neuropsychology, and behavior modification theories. In the next few decades, a greater emphasis on health reforms and technological advancements generated evidence for neural plasticity and functional recovery. Neuroimaging techniques with greater precision and acuity unraveled the mysteries of the human brain and provided greater insights. Assessment tools became more precise and standardized and encompassed a wide range of domains. Intervention techniques were made more unique, specific, and firmly embedded in theory. However, these advances gave rise to a number of questions:

- Should there be a standard module for a specific disorder or for each deficit?
- What is the ideal duration of intervention?
- Does improvement in cognitive functions translate to better daily living?
- What is the cost–benefit ratio?
- Are outcome measures ill defined?
- Should the frame of reference be the activity or the individual?
- Is there sufficient published material?

The authors consider these and a few other concerns as the impediments in the progress of neuropsychological rehabilitation. Each of these barriers with its influence on the field is discussed here.

## Approaches to Cognitive Rehabilitation

Since a majority of research in the area of neuropsychological rehabilitation has been done on patients with traumatic brain injury (TBI), researchers have developed a plethora of "retraining packages" for TBI patients. Although the interventions falling under the rubric of cognitive rehabilitation are heterogeneous, a consensus panel convened by the National Institutes of Health noted that these interventions share certain characteristics in that they are structured, systematic, goal directed, and individualized, and they involve learning, practice, social contact, and a relevant context [8]. Some of these are manualized, standardized packages that are available as ready-made solutions for TBI patients. When the authors read or hear about these, there is a sense of bewilderment because it challenges our basic notion that no two brain insults are the same and no brain responds to an insult in a similar way. Since each brain injury is unique in terms of areas affected and severity of trauma, it is erroneous to design standardized packages that would have little scope for customization. The authors propose that a rehabilitation program is most effective when it is tailor made to meet each individual's specific needs and is designed keeping their sociocultural context in mind. It is vital to assess comprehensively a gamut of cognitive functions and to develop a management plan depending on each patient's unique profile. Techniques should be designed keeping in mind the nature of the individual's deficits, and cognitive functions should be targeted in a hierarchical manner, progressing from basic to higher and more complex. Studies have shown that humans can be retrained in specific skills (e.g., learning to operate a computer, improving phonemic perceptions) after brain insults. The findings support the possibility of cortical plasticity throughout the lifespan for certain skills (not necessarily global functions) [9].

Similarly for other psychiatric and neurological conditions such as schizophrenia, stroke, and epilepsy, the clinician should assess the cognitive profile first and then sequentially target specific deficits. Though each disorder or syndrome shares a common set of symptoms and specific brain regions are known to be implicated, it is imperative to consider the precise manifestations and also keep in mind individual's sociocultural context when developing a module. For example, for patients from a rural background and with lower levels of education, computerized tasks should be avoided and task complexity should be kept low. The patient should be able to consider the task meaningful and relevant to his problem and context as that would affect his motivation and persistence in achieving set targets.

## Ideal Duration

Since there is little homogeneity in the treatment approaches used by clinicians across the world, it comes as no surprise when we talk about ambiguity regarding the ideal duration. Kwakkel et al. [10], in a meta-analytic review of studies demonstrating the efficacy of rehabilitation in stroke, reported that a statistically significant relationship was found between therapy duration on the one side and motor recovery and independence in activities of daily living on the other. Thus, the duration of intervention could be a nonspecific variable, thereby influencing the research outcomes of efficacy studies. Although it is widely known that learning and experience can stimulate changes in synaptic connectivity and plastic reorganization, there seems to be no clarity regarding the time of initiation, frequency, and duration of these learning exercises [11]. There are very few published articles discussing the role of duration of intervention in the rehabilitation literature; hence it would be premature to indicate with certainty its effects on the success or failure of an intervention module.

An issue of concern is the concept of "recovery" itself. Some theorists postulate that "recovery" starts after emergence from coma, continues at a gradual upward pace, then slows down and levels off, so that no more improvement occurs. The visual analogy is a geographic one—a plateau. This misconception leads families to despair when the rate of change decreases and causes therapists to terminate services when clients stop progressing. There is a tendency to "write off" clients when a first plateau has been reached. It is true that the most dramatic improvement does take place in the earliest stages followed by more gradual changes. However, the concept of the plateau is dangerous for two reasons. First, improvement following head injury is characterized by fits, starts, and bursts, often interspersed with periods of little apparent change, or even falling back. Head-injured patients are notoriously inconsistent in their progress at all stages. They may take one step forward, two back, do nothing for a while, and then unexpectedly make a series of gains. When one is preoccupied with watching for plateaus, it becomes easy to disengage from the client whose progress is sputtering. Second, long plateaus can be interrupted years later by energizing environmental events. The appearance of a new, committed counselor, or the increase in social contacts that come from being "forced" into a support group, can uncover functional potential in head-injured persons that has been dormant for years. Thus, successful rehabilitation of the head-injured person cannot take place until they and their family are aware of the new limitations, accept them, and formulate new goals based on changed expectations.

Duration of treatment has an important role in determining health insurance coverage and thus affects the feasibility and affordability of the intervention. The duration could vary from four weeks to four months or even more. In such a scenario, the costs to be incurred are difficult to assess at the outset of the intervention, and in cases involving law and insurance, such ambiguity could pose a daunting challenge.

Another related issue is that of providing home- versus hospital-based intervention. Considering the financial expense of providing hospital-based intervention, home-based cognitive rehabilitation programs could be assumed to provide some relief by reducing the number of hospital visits and the costs involved in seeking intervention. A single case study has shown the efficacy of home-based cognitive retraining in TBI. A 32-year-old male was referred for post head injury neuropsychological assessment and rehabilitation. He was given a six-month package of home-based cognitive retraining. The training was given by the patient's wife. The neuropsychological profile of the patient was compared pre- and posthome-based cognitive retraining. The preassessment showed impairment in frontal and temporal lobe functions. Postintervention results indicated improvement in cognitive functions, occupational functions, and social functioning [12]. However, an important limitation plaguing home-based interventions is the fact that caretakers often lack the professional expertise and skills required to modulate the tasks based on the patient's performance.

## Is Improvement and Generalization Just a Game of Numbers?

In order to measure the efficacy of any psychotherapeutic approach, it is essential that the gains made be substantial, enduring, and translate into functional skills for the individual. Some of the major criticisms of studies demonstrating the efficacy of neuropsychological rehabilitation include the time intervals at which the outcomes are measured. If the outcomes are measured too soon after the injury, it becomes difficult to distinguish between the effects of spontaneous recovery and the gains due to the rehabilitation program [13]. Another criticism that is leveled against the efficacy of rehabilitation studies is the nature of the outcome measure itself. Some studies have used the assessment measures only as the training tasks; hence any improvement on the posttraining measure could be considered a mere practice effect and is thus a false indicator of efficacy [14,15]. The litmus test for any rehabilitation program is the generalizability of the gains made in the clinical setting to patient's life situations.

A systematic evidence review by the Blue Cross Blue Shield Association Technology Evaluation Center [16] concluded that cognitive rehabilitation for TBI does not meet the Technology Evaluation Centre criteria. An important weakness in the literature on cognitive rehabilitation is that many clinical trials report impacts of cognitive rehabilitation on cognitive tests rather than on health outcomes. The assessment stated that "demonstration of the effectiveness of cognitive rehabilitation ... requires prospective, randomized designs that employ validated measures of health outcomes."

After patients undergo direct retraining for a cognitive impairment, final analyses often show only modest improvements on certain psychometric tests or tasks. Clinically, often the impact of an impairment-oriented approach on an individual's daily functioning appears minimal. Taking these issues into consideration, some clinicians emphasize that retraining should be done in the individual's natural context so as to provide functional skills and diminish specific barriers posed by the situation [13,17–19]. They assert that training in artificial lab situations does not translate well into enrichment in real-life situations. However, such a proposition challenges the behaviorist concept of "transfer of learning," which forms the core of human learning. In all forms of psychotherapy, the therapist's task is to provide the basic skills and the confidence to apply to those skills in various situations. The model of cognitive rehabilitation is based on improving basic and higher cognitive functions in order to enable the individual to think rationally, plan appropriately, and deal effectively with the environment. Hence, the authors propose that the individual's specific environment be kept in mind while designing the entire retraining program; however, the fundamental concern should be reducing cognitive deficits, thereby promoting functional independence and recovery.

## Economic Costs

Every intervention needs to be assessed in terms of its direct and indirect costs and benefits (Figure 9.2). In India, nearly 2 million people sustain brain injuries, 0.2 million lose their lives, and nearly 1 million need rehabilitation services every year [20]. By 2020, the incidence of TBI is projected to increase worldwide. The death rate is predicted to rise from 5.1 to 8.4 million, and TBI will be the biggest health-care burden on the society. A study done at NIMHANS [20] has reported that the majority of the families of injured persons incur an average expenditure of Rs. 5000 (sometimes reaching up to Rs. 100,000) during their hospital treatment. It is important to remember that this includes only direct medical expenditure; indirect expenses such as loss of work, loss of income, and other expenses are an additional burden. The total costs of TBI are enormous, especially for developing societies.

Having discussed the huge cost burden that brain injuries impose on society, it becomes crucial to develop rehabilitation strategies that are cost-effective. These interventions should be targeted at making the individual functionally independent and reintegrating him into the workforce of the community at the highest level possible. Thus, the rehabilitation should be holistic (improving physical, cognitive, social, and work-related skills), brief (reducing the cost due to duration of the intervention), and sustainable (gains should be maintained even at long-term follow-ups). The biggest obstacle to the progress of the field from its current state is the absence of specific, evidence-based, and results-oriented therapies. In most rehabilitation centers,

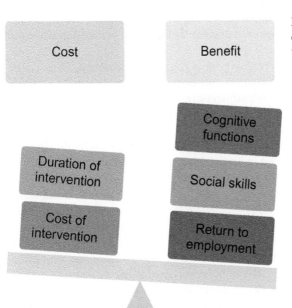

**Figure 9.2** Comparison of the costs and benefits associated with cognitive rehabilitation.

clinicians are experimenting with new strategies for each unique problem and learning from their experience. Considering the high economic burden that looms for the society with TBI becoming an epidemic, the need of the hour is briefer, more precise, and effective therapies.

## Ill-Defined Outcome Measures

A report of a consensus conference sponsored by the National Institute of Child Health and Human Development [8] concluded that, despite many descriptions of specific strategies, programs, and interventions, limited data on the effectiveness of cognitive rehabilitation programs are available because of the heterogeneity of subjects, interventions, and outcomes studied. An important aspect of measuring the success of any form of intervention is defining the outcome measure clearly and adequately. One of the major criticisms plaguing the field of rehabilitation in its current state is lack of a clear, specific outcome measure. "Improvement" is a subjective and qualitative term; for any field to be considered as a science, it is vital that it defines concepts objectively and quantitatively.

Outcome measures present a special problem, since some studies use global macrolevel measures (e.g., return to work), while others use intermediate measures (e.g., improved memory). These studies also have been limited by small sample size, failure to control for spontaneous recovery, and the unspecified effects of social contact. Researchers have emphasized repeatedly that a single outcome measure is not sufficient. Outcome measures should be multifaceted, covering a wide range of factors such as health-related, patient-reported, and general quality of life. Wade et al. [21] emphasize that rehabilitation research should have at least one aptly defined process variable and many primary outcome measures. To evaluate various novel approaches in the budding field of cognitive rehabilitation, one requires measures that are appropriate and sensitive enough to detect significant population differences in the process of recovery. Also, in order to compare the effectiveness of different approaches, it is essential that the same outcome measures be used in order to effectively compare two or more approaches and their impact. The authors of this chapter propose that the outcome measures be classified on three different levels (Figure 9.3). These three

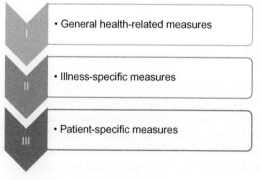

**Figure 9.3** Multidimensional classification of outcome measures.

- General health-related measures

- Illness-specific measures

- Patient-specific measures

levels of outcome measures should be consistently used across all studies to determine the efficacy of any intervention across a wide range of domains.

## Frames of Reference

The matter discussed in this section is in some way a continuation of the issue discussed above. The authors wish to discuss here the poignant points raised by Leonard Diller in his prestigious John Stanley Coulter memorial lecture (2004) on cognitive rehabilitation. Diller talks about "pushing the frames of reference" in conceptualizing cognitive rehabilitation from mere improvements in activities to changes in patients' subjective experience of reality [22]. This is an important aspect as it reiterates the need to look at the patient as an individual and not just a set of deficits that need to be fixed. When we deal with brain-injured patients, we need to remember that these are individuals who were functioning well before but have lost specific skills as a result of the trauma or injury. We need to be considerate of the sense of loss they have experienced, and in some cases the absence of this realization (denial) and hesitation in seeking help. Diller in his lecture quotes Goldstein's notion of health that goes beyond the absence of symptoms. It involves being able to accept one's reality by making efforts at overcoming one's difficulties through appropriate strategies.

It is imperative that, while evaluating the outcome of any rehabilitation program, one takes into account the experience of the individual himself. Improvement in scores on cognitive functions or other questionnaires does not necessarily indicate positive changes in a patient's subjective experience. Having an accurate sense of one's problems, setting realistic expectations, and making sincere efforts to fulfill them are important objectives that need to be attained at the outset of any rehabilitation programs. Experiencing a positive change in one's skills and abilities enhances confidence and reduces distress, thereby promoting health [22]. The authors in their setting use a visual analog scale as a part of their routine assessments at the beginning of any rehabilitation program. Patients have to indicate their subjective complaints and rate them on a score of 1 to 10, where 1 indicates minimum impairment and 10 indicates maximum. At the end of the training, along with other assessment measures, the visual analog is administered and patients are again asked to subjectively rate their complaints. The changes in the ratings indicate their experience and satisfaction with the rehabilitation program, thus yielding an important measure of its efficacy.

## Dearth of Published Material

Since the field of neuropsychological rehabilitation is in its nascent stage, it needs creative ideas and diverse thoughts from a variety of professionals involved either with patients or with research in this area. It requires a constant exchange of ideas and constructive criticism so as to escalate further into evidence-based science. However, one significant hurdle to its progress remains the lack of published material that facilitates the exchange of knowledge and developments. This occurs due to a wide gap between clinicians and researchers. Clinicians are involved with the process of rehabilitation at the basic level, but due to unexplainable reasons they are unable to share their learning and experiences. Researchers, on the other hand, examine the process from a distance, and in their obsession with objectivity, sometimes overlook the finer intricacies that are crucial to the process. For any scientific field to expand, it is vital that researchers and clinicians work in collaboration and achieve newer milestones.

# Future Directions

The aim of a good critical analysis is not only to identify weaknesses in a given field but also to provide a blueprint of suggestions that would help the field overcome its obstacles and grow exponentially. However, for a field that is expanding every moment, it is difficult to ascertain what the future holds. But as George Carlin wisely puts it, "There's no present. There's only the immediate future and the recent past." Hence, the authors wish to propose future directions derived from the limitations of the "recent past." Having discussed the current impediments in the previous sections, the authors would recommend the following guidelines for the growth of the field of neuropsychological rehabilitation.

## Research in Neuropsychological Rehabilitation

Research studies on the effects of direct retraining of cognitive impairments can be categorized into three broad types. The first includes retrospective clinical assessments of primarily neuropsychological and personality test scores before and after holistic milieu-oriented rehabilitation programs [23,24]. These studies are not randomized prospective investigations, and positive findings can be interpreted only as suggestive (not definitive) of their effectiveness. The second group of studies can be classified as primarily multiple individual case designs in which baseline, intervention, and postintervention assessments are made. Such studies often report modest improvements on certain target cognitive impairments. The third type of study is the traditional randomized group design in which subjects receive a specific treatment, no treatment, or pseudotreatment and are compared to control subjects [25]. These studies also tend to report modest improvements on complex tasks.

Considering the impediments discussed in the previous section (economic costs, skepticism regarding the efficacy of treatment, and lack of evidence), it becomes obvious that the first goal for the future is developing a strong scientific research base. It should meet the current standards of evidence-based medical research by using randomized control designs, using large sample sizes, and having double-blind participants to ensure objectivity. A few other recommendations could be as follows:

## Homogeneity in Population

In order to generalize the findings of a research study, it is crucial that the population should be homogenous. Only then could the changes be attributed to the effect of intervention. However, considering the fact that more rehabilitation studies are carried out in clinics or retraining centers, it becomes difficult to select samples that are completely homogenous. Hence, in such cases data could be analyzed using more robust statistical methods that could restrict the impact of sample differences on outcome measures.

## Application of Responsive Tests

Tests that are used to assess specific functions should be sensitive enough to pick up the deficits in these abilities. It is important that the tests used have good psychometric properties in terms of high reliability and validity, and the individual's performance should be interpreted in comparison to the given culture's norms.

## Accurate and Reliable Predictors of Functional Recovery

The terms "improvement" and "recovery" should be defined and differentiated adequately. The effectiveness of a therapy should be based on its outcome measures, which should be clearly defined at the outset. These measures should not be the same as the training measures and as far as possible should be parallel forms of the pretraining assessment measures. This would eliminate the practice effect and lend more empirical value to the data gathered.

## Brain Functional Imaging Methods

These methods have been virtually absent from the rehabilitation research scenario. With the advent of technology such as event-related fMRI, researchers can examine the impact of specific factors in the rehabilitation process. Also, the limitations of using the same assessment measures repeatedly, thereby leading to practice error, could be dealt with effectively [11].

Wade et al. [21] have emphasized four significant methodological issues that could be used as future directions in order to make the field more empirical. Figure 9.4 proposes guidelines that could be used to strengthen methodological rigor in the area of rehabilitation research. Empirical, continuous research forms the bedrock of any science,

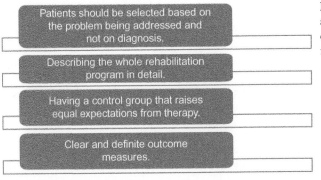

**Figure 9.4** Guidelines for a robust methodological design in rehabilitation research.

Patients should be selected based on the problem being addressed and not on diagnosis.

Describing the whole rehabilitation program in detail.

Having a control group that raises equal expectations from therapy.

Clear and definite outcome measures.

and in order to deal with the skepticism and controversy regarding neuropsychological rehabilitation, the recommendations discussed earlier are the need of the hour.

## Ethical Issues

Kirschner et al. [26] conducted a survey of 217 clinicians and admitting office personnel in an acute rehabilitation center, exploring the range of ethical issues faced by rehabilitation clinicians on a day-to-day basis. These are as follows:

- Health-care reimbursement issues such as concerns with insurance benefits for required services, helping needy patients, and ensuring continuity of care in the context of poor financial stability.
- Setting rehabilitation goals for patients, nurses, family, staff, physicians, and other rehabilitation professionals.
- Decision-making capacities of the patients, especially when they have fluctuating mental capacities.
- Confidentiality issues such as those that are sexual or aggressive in nature.
- Patient or family's refusal to accept clinical recommendations.

The respondents in the study strongly preferred interactive educational discussion formats for ethics education rather than self-instructional materials. In the future, specific guidelines regarding these ethical issues could be framed in order to ensure smooth functioning.

## Special Populations

Most of the rehabilitation literature has focused on retraining adult patients with TBI. Undoubtedly, TBI forms the major portion of patients needing rehabilitation; however, special populations such as children and the elderly have not been researched in detail. Most clinicians are in a state of perplexity when faced with children afflicted with TBI or elderly presenting with specific cognitive impairments. It would be enlightening to know how one could enhance functional recovery in a developing brain. A report that focused specifically on cognitive rehabilitation in children and adolescents concluded that clinical studies with designs capable of providing evidence for the effectiveness of interventions for children and adolescents with TBI were lacking [27,28]. The challenges of working with this population would be many, including distinguishing the effects of retraining from normal growth spurts and ensuring a regular, continuous form of intervention. However, the growth of the field would require its diversification into specialized populations and developing empirically based intervention modules for them.

## Expanding Horizons

A majority of research in cognitive rehabilitation has been done in the realm of TBI only. This may be understandable considering the frequency and intensity of this debilitating illness. However, for the field to advance, it is important that it expand its applicability and effectiveness in various other neurological and psychiatric disorders. A few of these important conditions are discussed here.

- *Multiple sclerosis*: Amato et al. [29] stated that despite its frequency and high functional impact, very little is known about effective strategies for managing cognitive impairments in patients with multiple sclerosis (MS). In an evidence-based review of cognitive rehabilitation for persons with MS, O'Brien et al. [30] concluded that cognitive rehabilitation in MS is in its relative infancy. Disease-modifying drugs may prevent or reduce the progression of cognitive dysfunction by containing the development of new cerebral lesions. However, rehabilitation is required to restore or compensate for the loss of functions. As for nonpharmacological interventions based on cognitive rehabilitation, few studies have used an experimental approach and, in general, results have been disappointingly negative. The authors noted that further research is clearly needed in this area.
- *Stroke*: Westerberg et al. [31] conducted a randomized pilot study of 18 stroke patients who were randomized to a treatment group (computerized training on working memory tasks) and a passive control group. More than one year after stroke, improvements were found in working memory and attention. There is some indication that cognitive retraining improves alertness and sustained attention, but little evidence exists to support or refute the use of cognitive rehabilitation for attention and memory deficits following stroke [32]. There is a need for better-designed trials of memory rehabilitation using common standardized outcome measures [33]. Several types of approaches are described, but their effectiveness at reducing disability and improving independence needs to be proven.
- *Brain tumors*: Meyers [34] found that the majority of individuals with brain tumors suffer from neurocognitive, emotional, and behavioral impairments that compromise their independence and interfere with their academic, vocational, and/or social pursuits. These impairments commonly include problems with memory, attention, and speed of thinking. Despite the often bleak prognosis and outlook associated with the diagnosis, many brain tumor survivors can enjoy improved levels of independence and functioning if provided with the appropriate support. With assistance from specialists in cognitive rehabilitation, brain tumor survivors can learn to use practical strategies that lessen the adverse impact of neurocognitive impairments on their ability to function in daily life.
- *Alzheimer's dementia*: Sitzer et al. [35] systematically reviewed the literature and summarized the effects of cognitive training (CT) for Alzheimer's disease (AD) patients. Effect sizes were calculated for 17 controlled studies identified through a comprehensive literature review. An overall effect size of 0.47 was observed for all CT strategies across all measured outcomes. The investigators concluded that CT shows promise in the treatment of AD, but further research is needed to evaluate the effect of treatment on function.

## *Educational Perspective*

Science cannot progress without scientists disseminating their information to others. This is partly achieved through training novices in the field with appropriate knowledge and skills. There is a dearth of trained rehabilitation professionals, and in the future, increased training would result in the availability of enhanced professional services to a larger population in need. This could be done in briefer formats of seminars and workshops or by introducing new courses and degrees exclusively in the field of cognitive rehabilitation. There is a pressing need to increase the health-care resources in order to impart quality services to patients afflicted with a wide variety of conditions.

## Prevention

The mark of progress in any medical field is when clinicians can shift from postacute management to prevention. Prevention of cognitive impairments is one area that needs to be explored, discussed, and conceptualized. The term rehabilitation should not just be about improving the deficits; it should also involve prevention of the deficits in functions or abilities. Prevention is possible by identifying factors that make an individual vulnerable to impairments, and it can be done at both the individual and the collective level. For example, the preventive aspect of dealing with stroke at an individual level would involve identification and management of risk factors; at a collective level, certain policy reforms promoting healthy habits could be advocated.

## Culture-Fair Therapy

Cognitive rehabilitation is not a culture-fair therapy as it exists. Most of the current strategies are biased toward the literate, urban, and sophisticated population. As a result, they cannot be effective in fostering plasticity of brain in illiterate populations, which raises questions about their validity. In the future, attempts should be made to make the intervention techniques as culturally fair as possible. An important goal in ensuring their widespread availability to various strata of society would be to make rehabilitation independent of contextual factors.

Having laid out the blueprint for the future growth and enhancement of the field of neuropsychological rehabilitation, the authors would like to conclude by quoting:

*A journey of a thousand miles begins with a single step.*

*Lao Tzu*

# References

[1] Boake, C. (1991). History of cognitive rehabilitation following head injury. In J. S. Kreutzer & P. H. Wehman (Eds.), *Cognitive rehabilitation for persons with traumatic brain injury* (pp. 1–12). Baltimore, MD: Brookes.
[2] Prigatano, G. P., Fordyee, D. J., & Zeiner, H. K. (1986). *Neuropsychological rehabilitation after brain injury*. Baltimore, MD: Johns Hopkins University.
[3] Prigatano, G. P. (2005). Therapy for emotional and motivational disorders. In W. M. High Jr., A. M. Sander, M. A. Struchen, & K. A. Hart (Eds.), *Rehabilitation for traumatic brain injury* (pp. 423–475). New York: Oxford University Press.
[4] Gianutsos, R. (1991). Cognitive rehabilitation: A neuropsychological specialty comes of age. *Brain Injury, 5,* 353–368.
[5] Barsalou, L. W. (1992). *Cognitive psychology: An overview for cognitive scientists.* Hillsdale, NJ: Erlbaum.
[6] Witol, A., Kreutzer, J., & Sander, A. (1999). Emotional, behavioural, and personality assessment after traumatic brain injury. In M. Rosenthal, E. Griffith, J. Kreutzer, & B. Pentland (Eds.), *Rehabilitation of the adult and child with traumatic brain injury* (pp. 167–182) (3rd ed.). Philadelphia: F.A. Davis.

[7] Newcombe, F. (2002). An overview of neuropsychological rehabilitation: A forgotten past and a challenging future. In W. Brower, E. Van Zomeren, I. Berg, A. Bouma, & E. De Haan (Eds.), *Cognitive rehabilitation: A clinical neuropsychological approach* (pp. 23–51). Amsterdam: Boom.

[8] National Institutes of Health (NIH) Consensus Conference. Rehabilitation of persons with traumatic brain injury. (1999). NIH Consensus Development Panel on Rehabilitation of Persons with Traumatic Brain Injury. *JAMA, 282*(10), 974–983.

[9] Merzenich, M. M., Jenkins, W. M., & Johnston, P. (1996). Temporal processing deficits of language-learning impaired children ameliorated by training. *Science, 271*, 77–81.

[10] Kwakkel, G., Wagenaar, R. C., Koelman, T. W., Lankhorst, G. J., & Koetsier, J. C. (1997). Effects of intensity of rehabilitation after stroke: A research synthesis. *Stroke, 28*, 1550–1556.

[11] Robertson, I. H. (1999). Cognitive rehabilitation: Attention and neglect. *Trends in Cognitive Sciences, 10*(3), 385–393.

[12] Jamuna, N., & Shibu, P. (2010). Home based cognitive retraining in traumatic brain injury. *Indian Journal of Neurotrauma, 93*(7), 93–96.

[13] Katz, D. I., & Mills, V. M. (1999). Traumatic brain injury: Natural history and efficacy of cognitive rehabilitation. In D. T. Stuss, G. Winocur, & I. H. Robertson (Eds.), *Cognitive neurorehabilitation* (pp. 279–301). Cambridge, MA: Cambridge University Press.

[14] Butler, R. W., & Namerow, N. S. (1998). Cognitive retraining in brain injury rehabilitation: A critical review. *Journal of Neurological Rehabilitation, 2*, 97–101.

[15] Ylvisaker, M., Hanks, R., & Johnson-Greene, D. (2002). Perspectives on rehabilitation of individuals with cognitive impairment after brain injury: Rationale for reconsideration of theoretical paradigms. *Journal of Head Trauma Rehabilitation, 17*, 191–209.

[16] Blue Cross Blue Shield Association (BCBSA), Technology Evaluation Centre (TEC) (May 2008). Cognitive rehabilitation for traumatic brain injury in adults. *TEC assessment program*. Chicago, IL: BCBSA; *23*(3).

[17] Garner, S. H., & Valadka, A. B. (1994). Medical management and principles of head injury rehabilitation. In M. A. J. Finlayson & S. H. Garner (Eds.), *Brain injury rehabilitation: Clinical considerations* (pp. 83–101). USA: Williams & Wilkins.

[18] Guercio, A., & Fralish, K. B. (1998). Integration of cognitive approaches to functional rehabilitation. In K. B. Fralish, & A. J. McMorrow (Eds.), *Innovations in head injury rehabilitation*, Ch. 9. White Plains, NY: Ahab Press.

[19] Ylvisaker, M., Turkstra, L., & Coelho, C. (2005). Behavioural and social interventions for individuals with traumatic brain injury: A summary of the research with clinical implications. *Seminars in Speech & Language, 26*(4), 256–267.

[20] Gururaj, G., Shastry, K. V. R., Chandramouli, A. B., Subbakrishna, D. K., Kraus, J. F. (2005a). *Traumatic brain injury*. National Institute of Mental Health and Neuro Sciences, Publication No. 61.

[21] Wade, D. T., Smeets, R. J., & Verbunt, J. A. (2010). Research in rehabilitation medicine: Methodological challenges. *Journal of Clinical Epidemiology, 63*, 699–704.

[22] Diller, L. (2005). Pushing the frames of reference in traumatic brain injury rehabilitation. *Archives of Physical Medicine Rehabilitation, 86*, 1075–1080.

[23] Prigatano, G. P., Fordyce, D. J., Zeiner, H. K., Roueche, J. R., Pepping, M., & Wood, B. C. (1984). Neuropsychological rehabilitation after closed head injury in young adults. *Journal of Neurology, Neurosurgery & Psychiatry, 47*(5), 505–513.

[24] Prigatano, G. P., Klonoff, P., & O'Brien, K. P. (1994). Productivity after neuropsychologically oriented, milieu rehabilitation. *Journal of Head Trauma Rehabilitation, 9*, 91–102.

[25] Gray, J. M., Robertson, I., & Pentland, B. (1992). Microcomputer-based attentional retraining after brain damage: A randomised group controlled trial. *Neuropsychological Rehabilitation*, *2*, 97–115.

[26] Kirschner, K. L., Stocking, C., Brady-Wagner, L., & Jajesnica-Foye, S. (2001). Ethical Issues Identified by Rehabilitation Clinicians. *Archives of Physical Medicine Rehabilitation*, *82*(2), S2–S8.

[27] Carney, N., du Coudray, H., & Davis, (1999b). *Rehabilitation for traumatic brain injury in children and adolescents.* Rockville, MD: Agency for Healthcare Research and Quality.

[28] Chestnut, R. M., Carney, N., Maynard, H., Patterson, P., Mann, C., & Helfand, M. (1999). Rehabilitation for traumatic brain injury. Rockville, MD: Agency for Healthcare Quality and Research. (AHRQ Publication No. 99–E006)

[29] Amato, M. P., Portaccio, E., & Zipoli, V. (2006). Are there protective treatments for cognitive decline in MS? *Journal of Neurological Science*, *245*(1–2), 183–186.

[30] O'Brien, A. R., Chiaravalloti, N., Goverover, Y., & Deluca, J. (2008). Evidenced-based cognitive rehabilitation for persons with multiple sclerosis: A review of the literature. *Archives of Physical Medicine Rehabilitation*, *89*(4), 761–769.

[31] Westerberg, H., Jacobaeus, H., & Hirvikoski, T. (2007). Computerized working memory training after stroke—A pilot study. *Brain Injury*, *21*(1), 21–30.

[32] Lincoln, N. B., Majid, M. J., & Weyman, N. (2000). Cognitive rehabilitation for attention deficits following stroke. *Cochrane Database System Review*, (4)) CD002842.

[33] Nair, R. D., & Lincoln, N. B. (2007). Cognitive rehabilitation for memory deficits following stroke. *Cochrane Database System Review*, (3)) CD002293.

[34] Meyers, C. A. (2012). Management of cognitive deficits and mood disturbance. *Handbook of clinical neurology*, *104*, 363–369.

[35] Sitzer, D. I., Twamley, E. W., & Jeste, D. V. (2006). Cognitive training in Alzheimer's disease: A meta-analysis of the literature. *Acta Psychiatrica Scandinavica*, *114*(2), 75–90.

[36] Luria, A. R. (1963). *Restoration of function after brain injury.* New York: Macmillan.

[37] Luria, A. R. (1973). *Higher cortical functions in man* (2nd ed.). New York: Basic Books.

[38] Zangwill, O. L. (1947). Psychological aspects of rehabilitiation in cases of brain injury. *British Journal of Psychology*, *37*, 60–69.

[39] Goldstein, K. (1942). *After-effects of brain injuries in war: Their evaluation and treatment.* New York: Grune & Stratton.

Printed and bound by CPI Group (UK) Ltd, Croydon, CR0 4YY

08/06/2025

01896868-0007